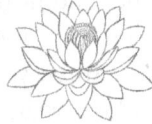

WHAT *Women* ARE SAYING

My husband and I had been trying to conceive for almost four years. It's been quite the journey with having multiple fertility treatments, several miscarriages, and lots of heartaches. When I found Shelly through a friend who has Shelly as a teacher, we had been on the journey for about a year and a half. Shelly has been with us since that time. She was actually the one to figure out that I had a thyroid issue (Hashimoto's) and worked with me to help get it in check and other various support measures. She also accompanied us to all our frozen embryo transfers and after. We are now mid-way through our pregnancy, and we are so excited! Thanks to Shelly for all her years of working with us and her support!

–A.R.

I'm so glad that I found Shelly! I saw her weekly for herbs when I had difficulty getting pregnant. The doctors wanted me to get surgery, but instead, she prescribed weekly herbal formulas, in combination with acupuncture, from the colleague who recommended her to me. It would have been more than worth my time and effort to feel healthy and balanced with the help from her treatments, which I did—but more than that, the docs were amazed my issues cleared up, and I had a completely healthy, uncomplicated pregnancy which culminated with the birth of my son. Shelly is warm, nurturing, and accessible—I always looked forward to our sessions, and I highly recommend her services!

–V. F.

For the past five years, my husband and I have made efforts to conceive. It has been a long and arduous journey for us. We have tried a lot of different ways to try and get pregnant since we weren't conceiving the natural way.

We both went to doctors to have our health checked out, and we were told we were fine. No red flags were evident, however, doctors immediately pushed me into taking hormones and going through intrauterine insemination.

For one year, I was put on Clomid, and nothing, no pregnancy. Each cycle was devastating and heartbreaking, but doctors kept pushing medication on me, and I kept taking it. After three years of attempting to conceive, doctors changed my medicine to Menopur, which is stronger than Clomid.

At that time, I also began to look at my diet and physical state of being. I reevaluated what I ate, changed my eating habits to a more vegan/vegetarian lifestyle, and began exercising, but still nothing. Menopur's effects on my body and mood were not great. I had strong mood swings and felt irritable and uncomfortable overall.

I wasn't feeling myself and was just not happy continuing to attempt to conceive the (Western) medical way. That's when I decided to look for alternative, more holistic-based methods and found myself under the thoughtful care of Shelly Tompkins.

I still remember the first day I walked into her cozy office and was greeted by her with a warm welcome. Shelly took the time to listen and read through my physical and emotional health history before starting any treatment. Once she had a profound knowledge of my health, she began healing and readjusting my body via acupuncture. I appreciate that Shelly not only took time to heal my body via acupuncture but also that, in every session, she took the time to understand my emotional well-being as well.

After three months of going to Shelly and also my doctor's visits, I decided to stop going to the doctor overall and simply continue acupuncture. Every week, Shelly worked on my body via acupuncture, herbs, and daily temperature readings. Six months after the first day I walked into Shelly's office, my pregnancy test read positive; you can imagine the excitement I felt! I am now seven months pregnant, and my baby and I continue our acupuncture visits with Shelly. I know that we are both under the best care.

This has been my journey. If I were to do it all over again, I would not go through any hormonal treatments via my doctor's office. My body and mind went through too much stress when I was going through that, and who needs stress when trying to conceive? On the contrary, if I were to do it all over again, I would focus on healing and readjusting my body via acupuncture, natural herbs, a healthy diet, and exercise. To Shelly, I am forever grateful.

–A. M.

When my husband and I decided to start trying for a baby, I was 35 and had been on the pill for many years. Shelly took the time to get to know me and my body and execute a plan for not only getting pregnant but my overall wellness. After a little over three months of seeing her on a consistent basis, I was pregnant and I felt fantastic. I continued to see her throughout my entire pregnancy and honestly had a wonderful pregnancy and birth. I am still a very happy client of hers and will continue to be! I cannot say enough good things about her!

–J. M.

After being told by a fertility specialist that I had almost 0% chance of getting pregnant on my own, we were headed down the IVF road. We decided to put it off for a more convenient time of the year to suit our busy work schedules and, in the meantime, see if we could make it work on our own. We immediately decided to go all in and do acupuncture as well. Shelly was referred to me by a family member. This was my first time doing acupuncture or any form of Eastern medicine, and in so many ways, it exceeded my expectations. I've always felt rushed at my regular doctors' offices and left wanting to ask more questions. I've never felt like that with Shelly. She asks a ton of questions, never seems rushed, and really listens to her patients. She is always available to answer my questions and has informative responses that I trust. Shelly is super friendly and cares deeply about her patients. I can also say that within two months of seeing Shelly, I conceived! I highly recommend Shelly for any fertility needs you may have. This is money well spent!

–M.V.

Conception
SECRETS

A Couple's Guide to Getting
Pregnant After Struggling with
Infertility or Miscarriage

SHELLY WEBER-TOMPKINS, L.Ac, CFMP

CONCEPTION SECRETS

A Couple's Guide to Getting Pregnant After Struggling with Infertility or Miscarriage

For permission requests, speaking inquiries, and bulk order purchase options, email shelly@shellytompkins.com.

Online storefront for herb/supplement orders: ShellyTompkins.com/products

Fertile Lifestyle Acupuncture and Integrative Medicine | **ShellyTompkins.com**

ISBN: 979-8-218-41015-5

Designed by Esther Moody

Edited by Mary Rembert and Lori Lynn

Photography by Monique Feil

"Most of the important things in the world have been accomplished by people who have kept on trying when there seemed to be no hope at all."

–DALE CARNEGIE

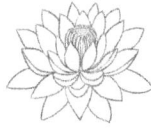

Contents

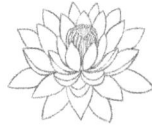

Dedication

This book is dedicated to all the women out there suffering in silence as they try to start their family. I hope this book will guide you in the next steps that will lead you to your goal. You are awesome and powerful, and I wish you the strength of heart to continue your journey.

THE

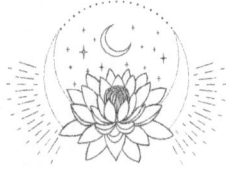

Beginning

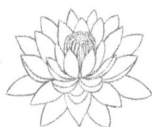

HAVING A *Baby* SHOULDN'T BE THIS HARD

All they wanted was to have a baby. For years, Kara and Jordan had been trying to get pregnant, but every year, they would find their hearts heavy and their arms empty. Why was it so hard for them? Wasn't it supposed to be easy to get pregnant in your 20s?

They thought they had tried it all. Hormone testing, sperm testing, intrauterine insemination. They were almost ready to give up when a close friend recommended my clinic. Knowing that other fertility specialists hadn't been able to help, they wondered how this time would be different.

As they walked into my office, they brought all their confusion, frustration, and despair. I could feel the heaviness in the room. Kara and Jordan were desperate and ready to do whatever it took to become parents—to finally have a baby of their own. After describing some of her physical issues, Kara opened up about what was going on emotionally. Sitting on her kitchen counter were not one, but *two* baby shower invitations. Both arrived in the same week.

Add to that the pain of seeing her friend's birth announcement on social media. She was exhausted from putting on a smile in front of everyone else. Even though she was genuinely happy for her friends (who seemed to have no trouble getting pregnant), behind closed doors, all she got was another negative pregnancy test. She was starting to feel betrayed by her own body.

While Kara was 25 years old, her husband Jordan was 31. He had type 1 diabetes and was on insulin. A hypothyroidism diagnosis had him taking levothyroxine. Due to his regular sports and gym time, he had back, hip, knee, shoulder, and wrist pain. He also had frequent headaches from clenching his jaw. He would still exercise every day, even with the pain. He struggled with insomnia and mental restlessness. When Jordan began working with me, we tested for male factor infertility. It's not just the egg; it's also the sperm that makes a good embryo.

Over the next seven months, as Kara continued her fertility-based treatments—acupuncture, herbal therapy, and vaginal steams—the vestibular pain she had been experiencing almost completely disappeared. Jordan had less pain and stress, and his testosterone levels increased without medication.

After seven months of treatment, Kara called me with the wonderful news. Her pregnancy test finally came back positive! Today, she and Jordan are proud parents of a healthy baby boy.

Kara and Jordan's story has a happy ending, but what if they could have avoided all those years of heartache? What if they had realized early on what was impacting their fertility?

----)) ● ((----

Another client, Anna, had also been trying for three years to get pregnant. She and her husband Bob had been to several doctors and done research and were trying to figure out why they couldn't have a baby, but they kept hitting a wall.

At 35 years old, Anna came to me physically and emotionally exhausted. Bob seemed mentally tired and disheartened. They had already tried three IUIs (in uterine inseminations) and two IVFs (in vitro fertilization). They didn't want to give up their dream of having a family, but they didn't know what to do next. Anna said I was their last hope.

After looking at their bloodwork and getting detailed health information, I helped Anna and Bob create a fertility plan that didn't feel overwhelming.

They agreed to follow the protocol, knowing there were no guarantees, but with renewed hope in their hearts.

Five months later—sooner than even I was expecting—I got the call I had been eagerly awaiting. Anna was pregnant!

Today, she and Bob have a healthy daughter and couldn't be happier with this beautiful addition to their family.

—))●((—

If you are having trouble conceiving, this book is here to empower you! It's important to know that infertility is not your fault. So many factors can impact fertility—a significant one that often gets overlooked is your partner! Male factor infertility is common and something that every couple who is having trouble getting pregnant should test for.

You can learn to be your best advocate by learning which tests to ask your doctor to order, understanding how those results can impact your conception, and, most importantly, having an action plan to make the necessary changes.

If this has been a long, frustrating, and disheartening road, please know you don't need to suffer alone in silence. I empathize with your struggle. I know what it feels like when the biological clock is ticking so loudly that you can't think straight, but conception isn't happening. If your partner is not "on board" with starting a family, it can add to the stress and angst you're feeling when you want to have a baby so badly.

When a friend tells you they are pregnant after you have been trying for a year or more with no success, it feels painful to your spirit. You wish them well and are happy for them, but inside, you are crying.

There's also the frustration of the unanswered reasons for not conceiving. You may have only been able to have a few basic tests done, if that, as to why you're not getting pregnant, only to hear, "Just keep trying." Unless you've already seen a fertility specialist, sperm, egg, and hormone testing are not typically offered by your M.D.

You need these answers to fix whatever is holding up your progress. The clock only seems to tick louder each month or year that you don't conceive, or if you do conceive, maybe you're having difficulty holding your pregnancy.

Trying over and over without making any changes can be the recipe for insanity or anxiety. However, knowing what to change is hard if you don't find the problem! Learning what could be delaying your conception or causing a miscarriage is the first step. Then, being willing to follow a plan that can make a difference and sticking with it is a huge and very important part of success with everything, including conception.

I also want to clarify that sometimes an IUI or IVF is the best and only option for some couples. I will walk you through all the areas that can interfere with conception and what to do, as well as steps to take if IVF is your best option. In the last section, I will discuss finding a good fertility specialist if you find that you need one.

Unfortunately, the statistics show the number of those dealing with infertility is growing yearly, as more and more couples are having to seek out experts after many months or years of trying without understanding why it's not working.

Infertility, defined as not being able to get pregnant after one year of trying, is more common than most people know, as many won't talk about it with their family or friends. Often, they won't admit that they're "trying," preferring to wait until they do conceive and get past the first trimester before sharing the good news.

It can be an emotional time, especially if you have had a miscarriage or there is continued fear and grieving from having experienced a stillbirth.

Most couples also experience family pressure or well-meaning friends asking, "When are you going to start a family?" Unfortunately, most people don't realize how emotional this line of questioning is for those who have been trying for a while without success.

I understand the pain firsthand and wrote this book specifically for *you*.

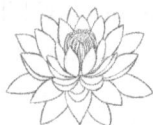

WHO IS
Shelly TOMPKINS?

Before starting my acupuncture practice in Chinese medicine and then studying functional medicine, I struggled with infertility. I vividly remember the feelings when a good friend got pregnant—especially when they weren't even trying! I remember saying, "Congratulations, I'm so happy for you!" and then going into the bathroom and bawling my eyes out, feeling the grief so acutely that it was like a physical punch in my gut.

The emotional roller coaster and the angst were present all the time. I could hear the clock ticking—it was so loud in my head.

Women who were on the same journey started coming into my practice. I found that I had so much empathy for couples who were trying to conceive. Throughout my career, I've also met and helped many couples and held their hands through this tumultuous time.

Nine years after starting my acupuncture practice, I had a revelation. Even though I see patients aged 12 to 92, my practice shifted to focusing more on my true passion: helping families grow.

I was seeing more and more women and couples who needed help conceiving and navigating the tricky waters of fertility treatments. Infertility was not a common specialty when I began my Chinese medicine career, but I devoured every bit of Chinese medicine wisdom I could find. More than 35 years later, I still obsess over learning everything I can about natural fertility!

I learned how Chinese medicine could help regulate menstrual cycles, balance hormones, and provide a beautiful foundation for a healthy pregnancy.

Sometimes, we were successful; other times, things were more complicated. A simple question haunted me: "Why do acupuncture and herbs help most of my patients get pregnant, but not all?" "I'm not sure" was not good enough for my inquisitive mind! While I was confident in the power of Chinese medicine, I knew I needed to dive deeper into their health and genetics.

I discovered a new field of innovative, natural medicine through my fertility studies: functional medicine. I knew that this field would allow me to help my patients conceive and hold a pregnancy, as the lab testing would give me more information on which factors were impacting their efforts so I could address them.

I studied with expert doctors to understand and prescribe a wide range of lab and hormone tests. I learned a new way to look at the body, medicine, and diet. With an even greater understanding of the reproductive system, I was able to finally understand why some of my patients weren't conceiving—and which steps would lead to better success.

Chinese and functional medicine work *perfectly* together to enhance the body's ability to conceive by creating a healthy, fertile environment. This comprehensive approach starts with helping couples conceive and then continues with family care into perimenopause and menopause.

I had a 40-year-old patient who had been trying to get pregnant for years. We had been working together for months and months to get her body healthy and increase her chances of getting pregnant.

One day, she texted me and said that her doctor had sent her an HCG report, and she had no idea what the numbers meant. I took one look at the report, and I was overjoyed! I got to be the one to tell her that she was pregnant! She had a healthy baby and went on to have another one naturally a year later.

These moments make this all worthwhile—the joy of helping a couple fulfill their heart's desire to become parents. After years of treating couples with infertility, I want to share what I wish I could have recommended to all my patients years before they began trying to conceive—discuss the most important steps to take now to become your most fertile so that you not only conceive but also maintain the pregnancy.

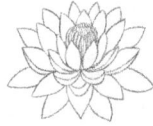

WHO THIS
Book IS FOR

Many women come into my practice thinking things like …

- If I'm having a period, I must be ovulating.
- If I have a 28-day cycle, I must be ovulating on day 14.
- He's young, so his sperm must be fine.
- All prenatal vitamins are equally good for me.
- It's usually the woman who has the fertility issue.
- High stress and lack of sleep don't affect fertility.
- If I've had a child before, I should be getting pregnant easier this time.
- Drinking 4-5 cocktails a week shouldn't mess with fertility.
- If the OPK (ovulation predictor kit) says that I ovulated on day 8, I can't have another LH spike.

The truth is all of these ideas are myths and misconceptions. So much misinformation gets circulated by our well-meaning family and friends, popular culture, social media, and faulty websites … It's hard to know what to believe and what course to take to get from where you are (struggling with infertility) to where you want to be (the proud mama of a beautiful, healthy baby)!

If you feel like you've tried everything or you're just now thinking about starting a family, you're in the right place. The best time to begin preparing for a baby is months before conception. And if you start now, your chances of being able to celebrate with a gender-reveal party or sending out birth announcements will go up exponentially.

I wish I could tell you that my story included all of those joys, but the truth is, I didn't have a supportive partner. So, instead of getting pregnant, I got a divorce. But because I know first-hand the longing for a child of your own, I have deep empathy for the women who reach out to me for help.

As countless women get healthy and strong so they can get pregnant and carry a baby to term, I know I'm doing the work I was meant to do. And every time I get a call saying, "I'm pregnant!" my heart overflows with joy.

There is no greater honor for me than to be part of helping you experience your heart's desire. On the other side of this path, you will discover a version of yourself that is beautiful, capable, healthy, strong, and worthy of all the good things this life has to offer.

The first step is to decide. Are you ready to do what it takes? If you're ready, then let's travel this road together. Remember, you are worthy, and you are not alone.

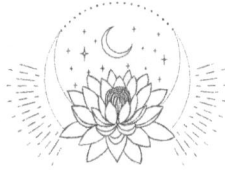

CREATING
Fertile Ground
FOR CONCEPTION

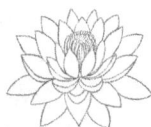

THE *One Thing* ANYONE CAN DO
TO INCREASE FERTILITY
(AND IT'S FREE!)

"I will not let the stress of
infertility overtake my life."

—ANONYMOUS

There's a lot more to Kara's story than I shared with you in the introduction. She and her husband Jordan had indeed tried for years to get pregnant. It's also true that after only seven months of combining Chinese medicine with functional medicine, they were able to conceive. But before that, 25-year-old Kara had been suffering in silence.

She was dealing with a host of different symptoms, including acne, painful periods, and chronic pain in and around her vagina (a condition called vestibulodynia). She described her discomfort as more of a burning, stinging sensation with intermittent pain. She found that wearing tampons during her period caused even more pain. Her cycle lasted three to seven days with light flow and spotting.

I asked a series of questions and discovered that she was following a vegan diet and had problems with her digestion and with frequent gas and bloating. She didn't typically drink enough fluids, as she couldn't take many bathroom breaks at work.

Her body felt cold, including her hands and feet. She also had a stressful job. Her energy level was good until midday, and then she would feel tired for the rest of the day, with no problems with her sleep.

Hormone testing showed that she was low on free testosterone, so her doctor had given her topical testosterone cream to put on the vulva to help the imbalance of hormones and for the pain. The testosterone cream caused her to have acne and clumpy vaginal discharge.

I suggested that she stop the topical testosterone cream for the time being and recommended weekly acupuncture treatments to regulate her hormones. During these sessions, I used heat lamps to warm her body and recommended more cooked foods and warm drinks in her diet to help with her digestion.

She came in for bi-weekly yoni (vaginal) steams between the end of her cycle and ovulation to help blood circulation and healing to her vulva/vagina.

I also recommended an herbal blend to increase blood and fluids to her reproductive system (specifically the vulva and to address the vestibulodynia) and a chlorophyll liquid to add to water and drink daily to build her blood levels.

All of these changes helped to decrease her pain, which ended up lowering her stress. By changing her diet, she was able to reduce the inflammation in her body. In addition, the herbs and treatments added moisture and good cervical mucus, which she had been lacking when she came in to see me.

She was happy with the changes and encouraged that her pain was decreasing quickly and she was having better cervical mucus at ovulation.

Because I understand that difficulty conceiving involves both partners, I also saw Kara's husband, Jordan. He was taking a men's multivitamin, an omega-3-turmeric blend for inflammation, and a supplement for adrenal support. I recommended weekly acupuncture treatments to reduce pain and inflammation, which are stressors.

Constant stress can increase cortisol levels, so they aren't creating reproductive hormones. We worked on hormone regulation and supporting his kidneys/adrenals/thyroid from the effects of stress.

Jordan's testosterone increased naturally as his stress decreased. Reducing Jordan's stress directly impacted his pain levels. And when Jordan and Kara began to find freedom from pain, they started enjoying each other more. Their collective stress as a couple went down, and their fertility went up.

Today, they have a healthy baby boy and the new stress that comes with caring for a newborn baby, but now they have the tools to manage their day-to-day stress, and their little family is thriving.

I am often amazed at how much of a part stress plays in preventing couples from getting (and staying) pregnant and delivering healthy babies.

Anxiety, depression, and relationship issues are common when facing infertility challenges. Friends and family can often say things they think are helpful, but they sound patronizing and hurtful, revealing their lack of understanding of your feelings around the subject.

This is why I suggest finding either a fertility counselor or a fertility group where you can discuss your thoughts and feelings, not only without judgment but, more importantly, with thoughtful steps and ideas on how to be gentle with yourself and build a mental space of peace and understanding for you and your partner.

This book covers many physical aspects of fertility, but no one knows what you're going through on an emotional level better than you. If you're struggling, I urge you to talk to someone. With telemedicine being so much more available, you can find someone local or in another state to help you.

WORK TOGETHER AS A COUPLE

- Two-way communication is vital. Try using "I feel" when sharing thoughts or addressing concerns so you can listen to each other without creating blame.

- If communication often feels problematic, consider couples therapy to work on better ways to talk to each other about your needs and concerns.

- Have a date night and make time for each other at least two times a month.

- Make love on nights other than when you're ovulating, and try to keep it fun. If it's always about trying to make a baby, the stress could begin to make intimacy feel like a chore.

- Remember, when you are sick or tired, sperm and eggs might not be at their peak. Give yourself a break and rest instead.

- Think of ways to help each other, as this can create better communication, and you'll both be in a better place in your relationship to have intimacy.

I would also suggest that you each have time to yourself, so you have a relaxing break after working all day. Sometimes, not discussing fertility when it's really on your mind can be difficult. But each of you needs to have some "mindless time." Watch a game or TV, or read without feeling guilty.

I also bring up the need to appreciate each other's stress, as your partner may not always show how much it is on their mind. If your first words when seeing your partner are, "I'm ovulating now, let's go," remember that they may need to get into "home mode" first, even though they love the intimacy with you.

To help your partner get in the mood, give them 30 minutes of relaxation before saying anything. If you are having dinner first, make it a light meal so that you will both be able to feel passionate instead of sleepy! I know when you have the OPK with a smiley face, it's harder to be patient. But the more you work on relaxing, the better it will be for both of you.

I had one patient who already had two children but was having trouble conceiving a third. They wanted to add another child into their home, and it was a couple of years of struggle to make it happen.

She was very tired from being a "soccer mom," running the kids to school, doing several extracurricular activities that the kids were in, and taking care of the home. She had no time for herself and needed help to have a third, so she came to see me.

I told her that she needs to have something she loves doing, whether dancing, singing, boxing, or playing a sport. For her, the one thing that she missed the most was her art. She'd put that aside, feeling that she didn't have time. It had been several years since she'd picked up a paintbrush.

Even with all of the nourishing foods, herbs, and acupuncture she'd received, she needed to get back to something that she loved doing that "fed her soul." Adding art back into her life was the missing piece of the puzzle. She needed that "creation" aspect.

She needed to get back to her creative self and take time to draw and paint again to help boost her spirit to conceive. There is great value in taking time to do what you love. Feeding your soul is good "juju."

STRESS REDUCTION IS NECESSARY!

Finding ways to combat both you and your partner's stress is important. You both want to be in your best health when trying to conceive, and if stress factors are high and plentiful, it can lead to fewer hormones activating good fertility for both of you.

Trying to conceive when you both thought it would be an easy goal can be very stressful in a couple's relationship. Kind communication is very important. Men may be more vulnerable if they are having sperm-related issues, depleted hormones, or even ill health.

Women also take on quite a bit of stress when they're trying to conceive, either with health issues, frustration with their body, or an inability to speak with their partner in a way that doesn't cause more stress in the relationship.

Stress factors broadly fall into four types or categories:

1. Physical Stress
2. Psychological Stress
3. Psychosocial Stress
4. Psychospiritual Stress

Look at each of these and see how many types of stress you might be experiencing. Ineffectively managed stress can take a toll on the body when stress-related feelings, moods, and emotions are pushed into it (usually termed psychosomatic).

Symptoms can include headaches, heart palpitations, fatigue, nausea, physical/cognitive/emotional pain and suffering, constricted throat and shallow, constricted breathing, clammy palms, anxiety, allergies, asthma, autoimmune syndromes, high blood pressure, and stomach issues such as upset stomach, ulcers, and heartburn and reflux.

Prolonged stress can suppress your immune system and increase susceptibility to infectious and immune-related diseases and cancer. Emotional stress can also result in hormonal imbalances (adrenal, pituitary, thyroid, etc.) that further interfere with healthy immune functioning and hormone production.

We all need downtime, but if there is a pattern of many of these stressors occurring, then it's time to look at what needs to change so that your health and fertility are not becoming impaired.

Unfortunately, there are times when trying to conceive starts to feel like a chore for both of you, and that can be a big problem, especially when stress is already a factor. Date nights or having activities outside of sex where you can talk, laugh, and regroup are important. Remember that you are in this together.

Remind yourself that you are a team, a loving couple that wants to add to the family.

The more you stress about what hasn't happened yet, the more it can affect your reproduction. It's a self-perpetuating circle:

- Chronic stress and anxiety can lead to hormonal disruption.
- Chronic stress increases cortisol levels that don't just affect your immune system.
- The more a person creates high cortisol levels, the more it will take away from the normal production of fertility-related hormones.

The important thing to realize with this section is that sometimes you don't realize that your stressors are more significant than you think, and you need to do something daily to balance your nervous system and find your center.

Usually, cortisol should peak in the morning to enable you to wake up and get going for the day. Cortisol is also there when you need a quick burst to your extremities for fighting or running.

A stressful situation can trigger a cascade of stress hormones that trigger your fight-or-flight response. The sympathetic nervous system functions like stepping on the gas pedal in a car, revving it up, and accelerating to avoid danger.

This hormone travels to the adrenal glands, prompting them to release cortisol. If you constantly feel in danger or overwhelmed, your body will overproduce cortisol, putting you in an unbalanced (low fertile) hormonal state.

On the other end of the spectrum, the parasympathetic nervous system is responsible for the body's rest and digestion response, referred to as feed and breed, when the body is relaxed, resting, or feeding.

It undoes the effects of the sympathetic nervous system after a stressful situation. The parasympathetic nervous system decreases respiration and heart rate and increases digestion.

The following techniques can minimize stress and get you into "feed and breed" mode!

- Slow, deep breathing of fresh air daily.
- Spend time in nature, take your shoes off, and feel the ground under your feet.
- Having playtime, especially with animals, as they have a soothing effect on us.
- Dancing and/or listening to relaxing or fun, upbeat music.
- Meditation and/or prayer, even for short periods.
- Laughing! Watch funny movies or shows, and tell jokes (deep belly laughs are great for circulation into our reproductive area).
- Walk barefoot on the grass; it's "grounding," literally.
- Deep gargling, humming, loud singing, and hot and cold showers can also help reverse the "fight-or-flight" response and switch you into parasympathetic "feed and breed."
- Daily affirmations for fertility.

Daily affirmations can be powerful since negative self-talk is rampant in our lives. Focus on the good and positive you deserve, which will feed your spirit. There are a lot of fertility affirmations online; pick what feels right for you and say it often throughout the day.

Affirmations can be a powerful way to reset your negative internal voice and fears. The idea is that you keep saying them until you believe the message.

Here is a positive affirmation for fertility: "I'm worthy of the very best of life, and I now lovingly allow myself to accept it."

You could also say, "All is well in my world. Everything is working out for my highest good. Out of this situation, only good will come. I am safe."[1]

Make time to breathe, take in the beauty, have some laughter therapy, and dance as if no one is watching. Be creative, draw, paint, mold clay or play-dough, whatever awakens your creative juices.

While reducing stress is a key component on the road to fertility, there are many other types of treatments that can help increase fertility rates.

ACUPUNCTURE AND ASIAN MEDICINE

Asian Medicine has been used for thousands of years to help regulate the body, resolve health issues, and relieve pain. Acupuncture involves using very thin sterile needles, which are inserted into points along meridians that run on the body's surface. Each meridian has these "points" that can help stimulate movement, aid circulation, and lower inflammation.

Every organ system has its own channel pathway that acupuncture can regulate. For example, a channel runs down the center line of the front of the body with points that help stimulate and regulate the reproductive organs to help conditions that affect fertility. These channels branch into the reproduction organs that are used to help with fertility and other conditions that both women and men experience.

A fertility specialist told one patient that I've seen in the past that her ovaries looked like "shriveled up raisins," and the only way that she'd be able to conceive would be through IVF. This patient decided to try acupuncture first to see if it could help. I'm so glad that she did, as within three months of weekly acupuncture treatments and herbs, she got pregnant naturally.

I'm not saying that everyone can become pregnant with acupuncture, as some genetic conditions, blockages, or scar tissue may not respond to treatment. Still, more people should know that acupuncture and herbal medicine are good first options.

Fertility conditions commonly treated with acupuncture:

> Female: Implantation issues, hormonal imbalance (ex: FSH or AMH are too high or too low, progesterone and/or estrogen insufficiency, androgen too high, etc.), poor egg quality, insufficient cervical mucus, luteal phase defect, PMS, menstrual pain, amenorrhea, PCOS, endometriosis, uterine fibroids, ovarian cysts.

> Male: Poor sperm morphology, low sperm count, poor motility, agglutinizing sperm, low libido, and more.

ASIAN HERBAL MEDICINE

Asian herbal medicine has a rich history spanning over 2,000 years, with its origins tracing back to ancient Chinese and other East Asian traditions.

The utilization of natural remedies is well known for its ability to help a wide range of health concerns, including infertility in both men and women.

This system uses a holistic approach, aiming to restore balance and harmony within the body. Unlike Western medicine's focus on treating specific symptoms, Asian herbal formulas are customized to the individual. They look at the body as a whole and find out through questioning, palpation, tongue, and pulse which formulas will help their system become more balanced and well. This takes into account each person's different constitution, imbalances, and what may be the root causes of their health concerns.

Studies have shown that the appropriate use of Chinese herbal formulas can significantly improve fertility outcomes, with some research indicating a two-fold increase in conception rates within a four-month period.[2] Asian herbal medicine's versatility also allows it to be used in conjunction with conventional fertility treatments, such as in vitro fertilization, to enhance their effectiveness.

CUPPING

Cupping therapy is an ancient alternative medicine that involves placing special cups on the skin to create suction. The cups may be glass, bamboo, earthenware, or silicone.

Practitioners believe this mobilizes blood flow to promote healing. Cupping therapy can be an effective procedure for treating infertility, too. In women, it is beneficial for several health problems like muscle tension, stress, hormonal imbalance, depression, polycystic ovarian syndrome, endometriosis, pelvic congestion, and menstruation irregularities.

INFRARED THERAPY

Near-infrared light therapy for fertility increases ATP (cellular energy production), thus improving egg quality, reducing inflammation, and improving uterine lining. Red light therapy helps improve sperm motility and quantity while decreasing abnormal sperm.

Red and near-infrared light therapy can work directly on the mitochondria, improving function and reducing issues like DNA mutations. This explains why a study from Denmark showed that two-thirds of women who previously had failed IVF cycles achieved a successful pregnancy (even natural pregnancies) with light therapy.[3]

YONI STEAMING

Yoni steaming, also called vaginal or pelvic steaming, is a natural and gentle way to help encourage pelvic healing for women.

- Yoni steams are gentle, restorative steam baths for the vaginal canal.
- During a yoni steam, you relax your pelvis over a bowl of steaming herbal-infused tea and rest while the medicinal steam encourages healthy circulation, warmth, and rejuvenation in the entire pelvic region.

There are different options for yoni steaming. You can purchase a larger type of bowl to squat or use your commode to place the bowl in, and you'd just set over the steam (make sure that it's not too hot). See the Resources section at the end of the book for information on how to do these at home. There are also boxes that you can purchase on sites such as Etsy that are pretty and reasonably priced, depending on the wood used.

Yoni steams are deeply therapeutic and beneficial for many women. These are the most common benefits of yoni steaming:

- Enhances Fertility—In Chinese medicine, fertility is often hindered by stagnation or coldness in the reproductive organs. Yoni steaming charges the entire pelvic region with warmth and circulation and sets a beautiful foundation for fertility.
- Relieves Pelvic Pain—Dysmenorrhea, menstrual cramping, and pelvic pain are the side effects of poor pelvic circulation. Using yoni steaming, you can bring healthy circulation and pain relief directly to your reproductive organs.
- Corrects Vaginal Imbalances—Women suffering from imbalances like candida, bacterial vaginosis, hormone imbalances, or dryness can find relief and support with specialized vaginal steams.
- Heals Vaginal Tissue—Postpartum or postmenopause, the vaginal tissue often needs extra care. Vaginal steaming is a natural way to directly nourish and stimulate intimate healing.

- Soothes Deep Emotional States—Even in healthy reproductive systems, yoni steams can encourage emotional healing or be enjoyed as a simple self-care ritual.

SUPPLEMENTATION

Supplementation of vitamins, minerals, and other nutrients is crucial in today's world due to soil nutrient depletion and heavy metals and pesticides in our food supply.

Modern agricultural practices, including the overuse of synthetic fertilizers and pesticides, have led to a significant decline in the nutrient content of the soil, which in turn has resulted in produce that is less nutritious than it once was.[4] Additionally, the widespread use of pesticides and the accumulation of heavy metals in the environment have contributed to the declining quality of our food, making it more difficult for us to obtain all the necessary nutrients from our diet alone.[5]

This is particularly concerning when it comes to infertility, which has been on the rise in recent years. Numerous studies have shown that specific vitamins, minerals, and other nutrients play a crucial role in reproductive health, and deficiencies in these nutrients can contribute to infertility in both men and women.[6] Supplementation with these key nutrients, such as folate, vitamin D, and antioxidants, can help improve fertility and increase the chances of a successful pregnancy.

Be sure to work closely with your healthcare provider to determine the appropriate supplementation regimen to address any nutritional deficiencies and optimize your reproductive health.

CHIROPRACTIC CARE

Regular chiropractic care can improve your breathing, blood vessel dilation, and digestion, all of which can potentially help a fertilized egg move through the fallopian tubes to the uterus. If one's pelvis is out of line, it can create pressure and cause stress on reproductive organs.

A twisted or misaligned pelvis can cause pressure on reproductive organs, potentially hindering the chances of conception. By addressing these misalignments, chiropractors can help reduce pressure on the pelvic floor and potentially increase fertility.

When choosing a chiropractor for fertility issues, it is important to consider their specialized training and experience. A chiropractor with additional training in fertility and maternity issues is better equipped to provide the best care possible for couples trying to conceive and continued care once they get pregnant.

CASTOR OIL PACKS

The potential influence of castor oil packs on fertility is not a new-age concept but is rooted deeply in traditional practices. Castor oil packs are believed to have several reproductive health and fertility benefits.

Some of the believed benefits include:

- Increased circulation of blood to the abdomen and pelvis to nourish the reproductive organs, among other things.
- Aiding detox by stimulating the lymph system.
- Helping the uterine lining for implantation and fertility.
- Improving egg quality and quantity and preventing too much thickening of the endometrial tissue.
- Relieving stress as it's also very relaxing.

Each of the following topics needs some weekly time to help you feel balanced and enjoy your time together as a couple. You want to feed your mind and take care of yourself; keeping these 12 areas in mind will help you stay healthy and can help your fertility as well: spirituality, creativity, finances, career, education, health, physical activity, home cooking, home environment, relationships, social life, and joy.

ACTION PLAN

- You should have a good idea by now (after PGS and lab tests are done) about which areas need the most support.
- Make sure that you're taking a good prenatal with folate.
- Antioxidants are key for chromosomal regulation, so ensure you're taking the recommended dosage. (Start with a CoQ10 and NAC.)
- Anti-inflammatories are important, so take a good fish oil (high in omega-3s and DHA). If you're vegan, using turmeric root as "golden tea" or grated fresh in foods and smoothies, as well as in pill form, can be helpful.

- For information on where you can buy yoni herbs and to consult on which tea might be best for you, please contact me at info@fertilelifestyle.com. See the Resource section on places to purchase a stool or DIY methods.

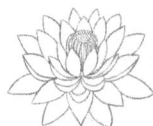

BY FINDING THE PATTERN(S)
THE *Solution* BECOMES CLEAR

"Infertility often comes with grief and loss.
You have to let go of the vision of how
long the journey will be and learn to flow
and become stronger through the process."

—HALLE TECCO

Remember Anna? She had tried multiple conventional fertility treatments before she came to me with three years of (very expensive) failed attempts to conceive. I listened to her concerns, asked more questions, and discovered some patterns that might be blocking her ability to get pregnant.

She worked from home and had low energy throughout the day. Anna had difficulty falling asleep at night, and her body was frequently cold. Her diet was pretty healthy, although she had some food sensitivities that she was trying to pin down. She had shorter menstrual cycles, typically 22-26 days, premenstrual breast discomfort, and cramps at a level-five pain (with 10 being extremely painful). She also noted constipation, had dizziness sometimes when she woke up, and her lower abdomen was cold on palpation.

Many of her symptoms seemed to indicate hypothyroidism, and I asked her to have her doctor check that as well as the marker for insulin resistance (HA1C). Her thyroid tests did show that her thyroid was underactive, and she was put on thyroid medication.

We created a food plan that she committed to, and I gave her some specific herbs to boost her blood levels and metabolism and bring more blood circulation to her reproductive organs. She came to me weekly for acupuncture and herbal medicine, and within five months, she and her husband, Bob, were delighted to see a positive pregnancy test. Finally! Their dreams of becoming parents came true.

In Asian and functional medicine, we look for "patterns" with those we help. Instead of treating one symptom as Western medicine often does (for example, if you have depression, you are prescribed Zoloft for hypertension, they give you Losartan, etc.)

All of your symptoms viewed together point toward specific patterns that indicate what organ(s) systems and gland(s) are out of balance and then decide which plan will have the best results.

The following examples show the most common patterns that affect fertility and normal menstrual cycles. They all have different options for herbal medicine, supplementation, diet, and lifestyle. It is a much more effective method.

Before I get into the patterns, I want to share why Asian medicine has a long history of helping men and women struggling with infertility as well as a vast number of other health problems.

Traditional Chinese Medicine (TCM) has a history of at least 3,000 years, starting from the early Zhou Dynasty of China or even earlier, as the oldest medical writings on herbs were found in the *Classic of Changes (Yi Jing)* and *Classic of Poetry (Shi Jing)*.[7]

These classics mentioned dozens of herbs in various situations related to healing and diet. Later, TCM evolved into an independent discipline as accumulated knowledge was documented in medical books.

While there are different branches of TCM, such as Chinese herbal medicine, acupuncture, and Qigong, the essential philosophy is the same. Western people might be most familiar with the metaphysics of Yin and Yang, representing the two ends of a spectrum: cold-hot, female-male, and inside-outside.

When this concept is applied to the human body, Yin and Yang are linked to different parts or organs of the body, or more simply, one's feeling of cold and hot. It is all about staying within the balance of Yin and Yang;

otherwise, falling out of balance gives rise to different syndromes or diseases. In such cases, herbs with "hot" properties can be used to treat a "cold" syndrome and vice versa.

This is a simplified view of a complex medicine that has helped so many people to find internal balance in all the organ and glandular systems of the body, including immune and lymphatic support and more.

With TCM looking at the body, the basis of treatment is about finding internal "balance" so that all systems can work together "in concert." If you only work on one area and neglect the other systems involved, your body will not find its balance; over time, the opposite can occur.

One example might be if there was too much river water running near a town, leading to muddy streets, mildew in homes, and sometimes flooding, then building a dam might seem like a great idea.

The dam would be great for a while until the day the town begins to run low on water.

It's not that a dam wasn't a helpful idea, but considering how the town will grow and need more water to support that growth, releasing or regulating the dam will be important to allow the town to flourish again.

THE PATTERNS OF INFERTILITY

Think of your body as though there's a concert always taking place within. Each instrument has a specific function, sound, and movement to contribute to the best music, all needing to be in synchronicity and harmony to make the most beautiful music. What we strive for in TCM and functional medicine is to ensure that the whole body has balance and is "in tune" to work together at its best.

We'll walk through pattern differentiation, keeping the whole body in mind, as over time, one organ system out of balance will have a domino effect on the others.

There are eight different patterns that we'll delve into that are seen with infertility and menstrual problems. Sometimes, it's one individual pattern involved, but more often, it is a combination of two to three patterns.

The first three of the eight patterns are classified as deficiency patterns:

1) Kidney Yang Xu

2) Kidney Yin Xu

3) Blood Xu

The last five are called excess patterns:

4) Liver Depression

5) Blood Stasis

6) Cold in the Uterus

7) Phlegm Dampness

8) Damp Heat

I'll walk through all these patterns in order with the symptoms as well as which diet and lifestyle changes can help best.

1. Kidney Yang Deficiency

Think of Yang as the furnace that fuels your metabolism or the catalyst that provides you with inner warmth and energy. When it's deficient or dampened, it doesn't help provide the energy and warmth your body needs in the luteal phase or the needed hormones. This is common with luteal phase defects, where there are issues with the embryo being able to implant.

With Kidney Yang deficiency, the basal body temperature stays low during the follicular phase (as is normal), but it doesn't rise after ovulation, as there's insufficient yang energy to do so.

Kidney Yang Deficiency Symptoms

- Scanty amount of blood (three full tampons or less for the whole cycle, or your period is late, or possibly none at all (amenorrhea).
- Feel cold all the time, bodily as well as both hands and feet.
- Cold pulling sensation in the lower abdomen and lower back pain.
- Pale complexion, without luster.
- Voiding a lot of clear urine, nighttime urination (may be frequent).

NOTE: These symptoms are often present with low BBT (basal body temperature) and hypothyroidism.

Ways to Warm Kidney Yang

- Eat cooked foods and hot soups and avoid cold or raw foods.

- Keep your liquids at room temperature and hot with herbal teas (Chai without caffeine or ginger tea, etc.)

- Keep your feet covered and warm (avoid walking barefoot on the cold tile, etc.)

- Choose warming spices in your food like garlic, ginger, and black pepper.

- Use a hot water bottle on your lower abdomen, lower back, and buttocks (this warmth can help open blood vessels to increase circulation into cold areas).

- Foot soaks before going to bed (this can be done with feet only in a tub, gradually adding hot water to warm water until it's tolerable. Do this every night, and it can help you sleep better too).

- Yoni steaming after menses are over, every other day until about two days before ovulation.

2. Kidney Yin Deficiency

Kidney Yin deficiency is a common pattern in women over 40. It arises from overwork and playing too hard, without time to rest and replenish the body, mind, and spirit.

Think of yin as the hormones that help signal the uterus lining to ripen and grow and the follicles to be well nourished. Diminished cervical and vaginal moisture are also an indicator of this.

Kidney Yin Deficiency Symptoms

- Menses may come early (before day 25 of your cycle) or it could be late with scanty red blood, without clots, or maybe amenorrhea.

- Dizziness.

- Blurred vision .

- Hot hands and feet, with intermittent sweating and/or night sweats.

- The tongue may appear redder and thinner.

Ways to Treat Kidney Yin Deficiency
- Stop all caffeine, stimulants, alcohol, and cigarettes.
- Rest and relax each day, get 7-9 hours of sleep (be in bed before 10 p.m.)
- Consume more root veggies, bone broth, soups, cooked vegetables, and balanced meals; don't skip!
- Avoid spicy-hot foods.
- No Bikram yoga or saunas (avoid excessive sweating).
- Don't overexercise (30-45 minutes max of moderate exercise).
- Meditation and stress reduction are important daily.
- Get grounded (step outside on the grass barefoot).

3. Blood Xu Deficiency

This deficiency is more likely if your periods are chronically heavy or if there's been trauma and/or surgery (where blood loss has occurred).

If blood deficiency signs are more severe, anemia can be checked by taking a complete blood count (CBC) test. Blood labs should include CBC with differential, iron levels, and B12 (methylmalonic acid via urine is the preferred test for B12 deficiency).

Blood Xu Deficiency Symptoms
- Menstrual blood may be scanty in amount, with pinkish-red blood, delayed cycles, feelings of fatigue, possible depression, or emotional (easy to tears). You may also feel dizzy, have a pale complexion, and possibly blurred vision or see black spots.
- Like Kidney Yin deficiency but without the heat and sweating.
- The tongue may appear pale and thin, like a pancake.

For treatment, follow the recommendations of Kidney Yin Xu. It is also very helpful to add more organic greens to the diet with this pattern. Liquid chlorophyll, taken two to three times daily, can also help those with anemia. This can be found at most health food stores. Try to buy it in a glass bottle, if possible, in order to avoid plastic.

4. Liver (Qi) Depression

Liver qi depression can manifest during different cycle phases. When the liver is more "stuck," it doesn't do all its jobs properly (the liver has over 500 jobs!)

This can be due to stress, frustration, environmental toxins, and more, which affect the liver's ability to convert hormones properly, which in turn can affect the pelvis and reproductive system.

Unfulfilled desires are a common reason for liver qi stagnation. It causes problems with the lining of the uterus forming and breaking down. A BBT chart may show a gradual fall in the first few days of your period.

Liver Qi Stagnation Symptoms

- Irregular menses (sometimes early, sometimes late).
- Dark clotted blood, and there could be cramping before the menses starts.
- PMS: painful breasts, depression, agitation, irritability; symptoms usually improve after the menses begin.
- Possible constipation at menses.

Ways to Help Regulate the Liver's Energy and Movement

- Foods eaten should be like the blood and kidney yin deficiency recommendations.
- Journal regularly to express feelings of frustration, depression, etc., to help with insights or ways to work through those feelings.
- Get some exercise each day to help lymph movement and blood circulation.
- Eat fermented foods such as kimchi, sauerkraut, and sour plums or season with umeboshi paste or vinegar.
- Utilize castor oil packs over the liver area when there are PMS symptoms.
- Try guided imagery and meditation to help reduce stress.
- Yoni steaming after menses, every other day until a day or two before ovulation.

5. Blood Stasis (Stagnation)

When the blood is thicker, possibly from lack of enough exercise or due to inflammation, the blood doesn't flow as smoothly through the vessels, which affects blood circulation that can cause pain, larger clots, possibly heavy bleeding or even blockage, where no bleeding is present. The endometrium, the inner lining of the uterus, is most affected by this pattern. Endometriosis, fibroids, PCOS, adhesions, and even cancer can cause blood stasis to occur.

Blood Stagnation Symptoms

- Menses: Irregular menses (sometimes early, sometimes late) often coincides with abdominal pain that is relieved by the passing of darker, clotted blood.
- Breast distension can be both before and during the menses.
- Fibroids, endometriosis, and other growth or adhesions normally fall under this category.
- The tongue may be dusky colored with purplish spots on the sides.

Helping Move Blood to Reduce Stagnation

- Follow the liver qi moving recommendations, as blood needs the liver's ability to support its movement through the reproductive organs.
- If there are feelings of cold in the abdomen or buttocks at the time of menses, applying heat can help the pain by opening up blocked circulation.
- Getting movement (at least 20 minutes a day pre-cycle).
- Avoid heavy-rich foods such as dairy, creams, sauces, and cold and raw foods, as they can interfere with blood circulation.
- Yoni steaming after menses, every other day until a day or two before ovulation. When TTC (trying to conceive), the yoni steaming herbs are recommended after menses have stopped and before ovulation occurs so as not to interfere with the luteal phase. But if you are feeling like a period is coming, and you are having any pain starting early without a positive pregnancy, a short steam with less heat could be utilized.

6. Cold in the Uterus

This pattern may be found in women who have never conceived. Cold tends to constrict blood vessels, so consuming too many icy drinks and raw foods or living in a cold environment can interfere with blood flow.

If the blood vessels constrict during your period, it can cause the period to be more painful, as you could develop clots that can be uncomfortable to pass. Also, a lack of good blood flow to the reproductive organs can negatively impact fertility. Fertility is supported by good blood supply and open circulation in the vessels so the ovaries can produce eggs and the uterus can build a healthy lining for an embryo.

Cold in the Uterus Symptoms

- Delayed menstrual cycles, scanty bleeding, and small clots.
- Painful menses that are relieved with heat.
- Feeling cool/cold during menses, especially the belly/buttocks.
- May have a pale-looking face, and a sore back and fatigue.
- The tongue may be pale with a thick white coat.

Ways to Treat Cold in the Uterus

- Follow the diet for kidney yang xu and the bodily recommendations for blood stagnation.
- Heat will feel good in this pattern, but pressure on your abdomen will not feel good (it feels good with deficiency, but this is more of a blocked feeling). Hot packs can be helpful here, especially before menses and when pain is present.
- Avoid sitting on cold surfaces. Take off wet clothing from the gym/pool as soon as possible, take a warm shower, and dry off well.
- Yoni steaming after menses, every other day until a day or two before ovulation.

7. Phlegm Dampness

This excess condition can be caused by several factors. One is due to a diet high in sugars, carbs, and processed foods, leading to higher fat stores in the body. It also can lead to fatty liver disease and polycystic ovaries.

The liver releases stored sugars for energy and converting hormones, but excessive fat accumulation can impair its function. When the liver can't process and break down fats normally, it can lead to the accumulation of excess fat, which may be stored as liver fat.

In Chinese medicine, those holding excess weight are referred to as having a phlegm damp condition. PCOS doesn't only happen in patients who are overweight or obese; I have treated lean women with this diagnosis as well.

Phlegm Dampness Symptoms

- Irregular menses (maybe early one month and late the next).

- Mid-cycle pain, more vaginal discharge.

- Long-term infertility.

- Adhesions may be present (scar tissue post-infection).

- Prone to weight gain.

- Feeling of heaviness.

- The tongue coating can be thick and sticky.

Clearing Phlegm Dampness

- Avoid greasy fried foods, sugar, sweets, fruit juice, refined carbohydrates, soda, milk, or dairy products, including ice cream, soy products, wheat, banana, chocolate, or nuts.

- No alcohol.

- Eating a lot of steamed or lightly sautéed green veggies (not uncooked).

- Some starches like yam or sweet potato are okay.

- Add more diuretic-like foods to your meals, such as alfalfa sprouts, parsley, radishes, celery, cucumbers, lettuce, and kelp (avoid kelp if you have been diagnosed with Hashimoto's).

- Yoni steaming after menses, every other day until a day or two before ovulation.

- If candida, bacterial vaginosis, or other type of infection is present, don't steam, or use a light steam with the Clearing Blend instead.

8. Damp Heat

This particular diagnosis is typically seen when pathogens enter through the vagina, urethra, and even the rectum. It can occur with STDs, candida, yeast, bacterial vaginosis, chlamydia, or even occur from not changing out of sweaty gym clothes or a wet bathing suit in a timely fashion.

This condition is often seen with pelvic and fallopian tube inflammation. Inflammation in either of these areas is not helpful to sperm or embryo and needs to be cleared out before trying to conceive, if present.

Damp Heat Symptoms

- Vaginal discharge that is yellowish, possible bacterial vaginosis, HPV, candida.

- Pelvic inflammation, prone to ovarian cysts.

- Possible blockage of fallopian tubes.

- Feelings of heat and mental restlessness.

- Tongue: has a thick, sticky yellow coating.

- Most of these symptoms occur when inflammation is present.

Ways to Clear Dampness and Heat (Inflammatory Factors)

- Avoid greasy fried foods, sugar, sweets, fruit juice and refined carbohydrates, soda, milk, or dairy products, including ice cream, soy products, wheat, banana, chocolate, nuts, and spicy foods.

- No alcohol.

- Avoid spicy hot foods or condiments.

- Eat a lot of green veggies.

- Add more diuretic foods to your meals, such as alfalfa sprouts, parsley, radishes, melons, celery, cucumbers, lettuce, and kelp (again, remember to avoid kelp if you have been diagnosed with Hashimoto's).

- Yoni steaming after menses, every other day until a day or two before ovulation.

Acupuncture treatment and herbal medicine are also excellent in regulating all of these patterns and are very helpful in regulating the reproductive system and fertility.

ACTION PLAN

1. Did you note any pattern(s) that are similar to what you experienced? You might have found two or three patterns that fit your symptoms picture.

2. Please write down in your journal which patterns fit you the most, preferably with at least three or more symptoms that fit with your cycle.

For example, you could have a combination of these three patterns: kidney yin deficiency, liver qi stagnation, and blood stagnation symptoms.

Symptoms might be when periods are late, with a scanty flow darker in color and small clots and night sweats. Before menses begin, there is breast tenderness and irritability, with cramps that proceed to the menses and continue past the third day.

In the above example, I have three possible patterns, so I would follow the top two (that have the most symptoms that fit you and stick with those two protocols).

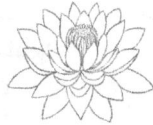

HOW *Planning* SETS YOU UP FOR *Success*

"A goal without a plan is just a wish."

—ANTOINE DE SAINT-EXUPÉRY

If you were heading out on a weekend getaway, chances are you would plug your destination into GPS and map out your route before hitting the road. In the same way, before you start down the road to conception, you want to consider potential obstacles and plan strategies in advance for success.

If you are considering starting a family soon, having a preconception plan is essential. In a perfect scenario, couples would take a year to get healthy, clean up their diet and environment, and complete basic testing. I know a year is a long time, but give yourselves at least three months to get on the best path to success.

I have compiled a checklist covering many of the areas mentioned above. Whether you are doing this with a partner or solo, there are important questions you should decide, such as:

- When do you want to have a child?
- Do you have a doctor who can do testing for you?
- Which tests do you need before trying?
- How much additional money will you need to provide for a baby?

- Do you have a designated room or space at home for a baby, or do you need to move?
- If you don't live close to either of your families, how can you manage funds for daycare before preschool or kindergarten?

I'm not mentioning this to stress you out. Quite the opposite. If you have a plan in place, then when you're actively trying to conceive (TTC), you can focus on being healthy for yourself and your baby.

Planning for work considerations is essential. If you struggle to find time to water plants, feed pets, and stay caught up with other everyday tasks, finding time for this and more when you have a child will be more challenging.

Start planning now what this will look like for you and your partner. In this way, being prepared can help lower the stress that TTC can bring.

Preconception health refers to physical, mental, emotional, social, and relational well-being before and between pregnancies. Health is not simply the absence of illness but a state where you have the necessary resources, community, and cultural support to achieve the best health possible for yourself and your family.

FERTILITY TESTING CHECKLIST

The following is the type of testing and screening that you'd want to have your doctor order for you and your partner. Blood tests are typically done for genetic testing and infectious diseases.

Genetic testing to consider
- MTHFR
- Sickle cell anemia
- Cystic fibrosis
- Thalassemia
- Tay-Sachs disease

Ruling out infectious STDs and viruses
- HIV
- Syphilis

- Gonorrhea/chlamydia
- Hepatitis C in those with tattoos and body piercings

ELIMINATING ENVIRONMENTAL TOXINS

Eliminating environmental toxins is crucial for women trying to get pregnant because these toxins can negatively impact fertility and increase the risk of pregnancy complications. We will go into more depth in Section 3, but here are key areas to consider.

- Quit smoking.
- Screen for alcoholism and use of illegal drugs.
- Occupational exposures—check with your employer for a list of potentially hazardous materials.
- Household chemicals—avoid paint thinners and strippers, other solvents, and pesticides.
- Radiation exposure in early pregnancy.

MEDICAL ASSESSMENT

Evaluate your health and dietary habits and what you can do to improve your health. Determine if you or your partner suffers from any undiagnosed or uncontrolled medical problems (such as diabetes, thyroid disease, dental cavities or gum disease, heart disease, asthma, hypertension, IBS, Crohn's, malabsorption issues, and sleep apnea).

- Diabetes—Rule it out, but if you are prediabetic, you'll want to make changes now.
- High blood pressure—avoid ACE inhibitors and angiotensin II receptor antagonists.
- Epilepsy—consider an increased dose of folate.
- Deep vein thrombosis (DVT)—switch from warfarin (Coumadin) to heparin.
- Acne—stop isotretinoin (e.g., Accutane).
- Depression, anxiety, and other mental health issues that are current—determine the benefits versus the risks of taking medication, as some of them can affect egg and sperm quality.

Many of these health-related concerns can be tested by your general practitioner (GP) and may depend on your insurance as to what will be covered, or you may be referred to an OB/GYN, urologist (for men), or a fertility specialist. If you are trying to get as much covered as possible by your insurance, get a referral from your GP.

Unfortunately, they may not be agreeable to all these tests as many insurance plans don't cover fertility. Finding an integrative doctor, functional medicine provider, or naturopath will give you more freedom to order these tests and to understand the findings and possible treatment needed.

Couples counseling is also essential, especially if there is already stress with communication between a couple.

It can be hard enough in a relationship during troubling times. If conception doesn't occur as quickly as hoped, it can strain communication, making TTC even more difficult.

Finding a fertility or marriage counselor locally or by telehealth can help. A good counselor can help you to use constructive versus blame-oriented communication with each other if conception doesn't happen as quickly as hoped.

Learning to talk to each other with understanding and care can go a long way in supporting each other when TTC.

I do feel that it is essential to understand the meaning of "unexplained infertility." In medical terms, the definition is "The diagnosis of unexplained infertility can be made only after excluding common causes of infertility using standard fertility investigations, which include semen analysis, assessment of ovulation, and tubal patency test. These tests have been selected as they definitively correlate with pregnancy."[8]

I believe there is always an answer to why conception hasn't occurred after a year of trying. Early testing can help clarify which issues need to be addressed.

You will learn about different health conditions that can impact the fertility of both men and women. I will walk you through the symptoms, testing to clarify, and healthy treatment options, as well as diet and lifestyle approaches that can significantly increase your overall fertility.

This is not a "one size fits all" approach. We are all different, so the steps that help you may differ from someone else's.

Most patients I see in my clinic are past age 35 and have been trying for 11 months or more before coming to see me. Some of these patients had already visited a fertility specialist to find out why they were not conceiving and may have already tried one or two IUI (in uterine inseminations) or had egg retrievals for IVF, but they weren't getting enough eggs, or the quality wasn't the best.

Since I'm an acupuncturist, I receive many referrals for acupuncture treatments from fertility specialists who have found them to be helpful for patients having in vitro fertilization (IVF).

When people are struggling to conceive, acupuncture treatment can help in assisting with IVF by helping to calm the patient and bring more blood circulation to the uterus. It's always my goal to help them conceive naturally before having to go that route, but sometimes it is necessary.

ACTION PLAN:

- Now is the time, before starting a family, to go through your checklist to consider your finances, living situation, and childcare needs so you won't have that stress during your pregnancy.

- Discuss which medical tests and screenings you will need with your doctor.

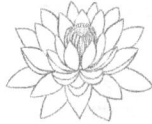

THE *Importance* OF HORMONAL BALANCING AND CYCLE REGULATION

> "I am equally blessed with love, harmony,
> and joy. I take in life in perfect balance."
>
> —LOUISE HAY

Susan's first menstrual cycle started around 16 years of age, with heavy blood and painful cramping each period. Her cycles were irregular, and she'd have lower back pain during her period. She took birth control pills (BCP) to help regulate her cycles, and they became more normal over the next year, progressing to a lighter menstrual flow by age 26.

She continued BCPs for 10 more years before stopping to try to conceive. Her body was used to receiving false hormonal signals because of the birth control pills versus her body making them. When she finally stopped taking them, her cycle and ovulation became irregular, as her hormone signaling wasn't regulating itself.

I have seen this same scenario with many women I have worked with over the years. They had started with birth control pills from the very beginning of their menstrual journey and then stayed on them for 10-plus years without a break. Long-term use, so early on, didn't help their body learn to make the normal connections with the reproductive system to make eggs and ovulate, so when they did finally stop the pill years later, it took more time to regulate their cycle and learn to stimulate the ovaries.

There are cases where pregnancy occurs within months of stopping the pill, but this isn't always the case. Hormone testing is a good idea a few months after discontinuing the pill. That way, the steps you need to take to become regulated will be clearer.

There are important and revealing things to consider with a menstrual cycle: the hormones that regulate it, the charting, or other tools you'll need going forward.

To understand this better, let's start by considering your menstrual cycle. This can reveal how well your hormones are regulated, if you have good blood circulation in the reproductive system, and whether any problems need to be addressed.

Were you on birth control pills in your teens to regulate your cycle?

If you never took time off from them before trying to conceive, and it's been 10 years or longer without a break, your ovaries may need some time to remember their job of ovulating correctly again. Everyone is different, but I suggest being off the pill at least a year before TTC if you've been on it for a long time.

How many days do you bleed each month? Less than three days? More than seven days?

This has more to do with how much blood you lose each month. If it's very scanty bleeding for the time that you bleed and you're not on the pill, you may need to check for anemia and/or check your hormone levels. You want to ensure sufficient blood to nourish an embryo and that you regulate your hormones to build a lining, with good luteal phase progesterone to help an embryo attach in the uterus and "hold."

How heavy is the blood flow?

If the bleeding is too heavy, it can also cause anemia or be due to a hormonal imbalance, so it's a good idea to have a vaginal ultrasound to rule out fibroids, polyps, or endometriosis if this has been going on for a while. If it's accompanied by abdominal pain, then endometriosis might be present and need more than an ultrasound.

What is the color of the blood?

You're looking for fresh red blood, not too pale or too dark in color, to ensure it's healthy, nourishing blood from which an embryo can grow.

Do you have sizeable clots during most of your periods (almond size or bigger?)

Small shedding of tiny raisin-size clots or threads isn't uncommon, but larger clots may be evidence of one or more fibroids or something slowing the passage of more blood that can form clots. This is where ultrasound is an excellent option to rule out fibroids, polyps, etc.

Do you have cramping that starts before you bleed but stops after the first day of real flow? Or does it continue and maybe become worse with the flow?

Out-of-balance hormones can cause this. However, if the pain worsens with the flow, there's usually more inflammation and possible clots. (It's important to get clarity on whether it could be endometriosis, fibroids, or something else so it can be treated before TTC.)

Do you have painful or sensitive breasts before your period or mid-cycle?

This usually occurs with hormonal surges you'll want to regulate before TTC. The smoother things go before conception, the more smoothly the pregnancy may be.

If you have PMS, does it last for a few days, a week, or more?

Hormonal imbalances or surges can lead to premenstrual syndrome (PMS), anxiety, depression, migraines, acne, and/or rage. Regulating hormones will help this.

With your emotions, do you find yourself sad or weepy before your cycle starts? Or do you notice depression, irritation, or anger before your period?

The same answer applies to the question above. Hormones that are not regulated can impact neurotransmitters that are involved with your emotions.

Neurotransmitters are chemical messengers that help nerve cells communicate with each other. They carry messages from one nerve cell to the next; the next cell can be another nerve cell, muscle cell, or gland. Without neurotransmitters, your body can't function properly. Some common neurotransmitters include serotonin, dopamine, and glutamate.[9]

Are your cycles regular (normally starting 26-32 days after your menses start)? Or do they start later than 33 days? Or less than 26? Are they irregular, and you're unsure when to expect your next menses?

It's good to have regular cycles, preferably between 26-32 days. The hormones are doing what they're supposed to do if the menses flow smoothly without pain or discomfort, your breasts don't hurt before or during, and your emotions are manageable without headaches.

All these symptoms and more can help you discover which issues should be addressed to help you conceive and have a family soon. Once the root issue(s) are understood, a plan with the best steps to regulate your hormones can be put in place.

We are looking for patterns with your cycle. If you know the pattern, you can find the best treatment! For example, if you have heavy periods, some noticeable clots, painful periods, or possible PMS symptoms (breast tenderness, moodiness, headaches, etc.), it may point toward impaired pelvic circulation that could, in time, lead to inflammatory issues such as fibroids, endometriosis, PCOS, and more.

There could be hormonal imbalances affecting the blood circulation through the reproductive organs and those that regulate your cycle and reduce inflammation.

THE STAGES OF FOLLICULAR DEVELOPMENT

Every stage of egg development, and that of the uterus's endometrium, depends on the right number of hormones being available when needed. Throughout your cycle, different hormones will be necessary in higher amounts. To get those hormones to the correct areas to help ovulation and implantation, you need specific hormones to be available, and you also need to have good circulation and blood flow to help them get to their destination.

These hormones are carried in the bloodstream to the ovaries in women and testes in men.

Good follicular development is essential, but so is being able to ovulate at the "optimal time of its development," as well as having open fallopian tubes and a healthy uterine environment.

What must happen to ensure that a good ovulation takes place?

- All hormone pathways must work well to send the correct signals to the ovaries to stimulate egg production and growth. Some reasons why this may not occur are luteinizing unruptured follicle syndrome (LUFS), PCOS, low estrogen levels, and even chronic stress.

- There needs to be free flow without obstruction in the fallopian tubes (no scar tissue, etc.)

- There needs to be enough good blood circulation to the ovaries, tubes, and uterus.

- Knowing the signs of ovulation's occurrence (we'll discuss BBT charting, OPKs, and what to note with cervical mucus.)

If you have irregular cycles, it is good to have your hormones checked, a pelvic ultrasound, and a hysterosalpingogram to rule out any strictures or other problems that could get in the way.

There are four key areas to measure with menstruation; the following note what is considered good:

1. Cycle and duration: 26-32 days, between Day 1 and menses beginning again with 5-7 days of blood flow
2. Color of the blood: fresh red to brown
3. Quality of the blood: not thick or thin, not clotted
4. Quantity of blood discharged: 50-80 ml total for entire menses

If you wonder how much blood period underwear and other products can hold, in a new study, Samuelson Bannow and her team tested 21 different menstrual products, including discs, tampons, pads, period underwear, and cups.

They found that menstrual underwear products were the least absorbent on the market, soaking up one to three milliliters of blood, depending on size. "Light" pads were slightly more absorbent, maintaining 3 to 4 ml. Tampons held between 20 and 34 ml, depending on the brand and flow rating, and "heavy" pads, which advertised 10- to 20-ml capacity, could hold up to 52 ml. Menstrual discs held the most blood—61ml on average—with one brand holding up to 80 ml.[10]

Menstrual Blood
COMPARISON CHART

BLOOD AMOUNT	REG TAMPON	MEDIUM PAD	DIVA CUP
1/3 FULL	1 ML	1ML	5ML
1/2 FULL	5ML	10ML	10ML
FULL	10ML	20ML	15ML

If you have had very heavy menses most of your cycles, it would be good to have your iron, RBCs, hemoglobin, and hematocrit levels checked by your general practitioner or obstetrician. The test that you'd ask for is a complete blood count (CBC) with serum iron, ferritin, and transferrin included. Anemia can impact pregnancy, as you need a good amount of blood for yourself and to nourish a budding embryo.

If there's a lot of pain with menses and/or clotting each month, then being checked for fibroids, endometriosis, or adhesions can help in understanding what factors may be contributing to inflammation and poor blood circulation and what types of therapy will help the most.

We will discuss helpful tests so you know what changes to make to lessen any factors getting in the way of conceiving.

HELPING OVULATION BE MORE SUCCESSFUL

It's important to understand the timing of ovulation, which is more difficult to do when cycles are irregular, too early, or significantly delayed.

The first thing you need to determine is why your cycles are irregular in the first place. Then, follow the steps to help regulate them and learn to recognize ovulation symptoms.

When I ask patients how they track their ovulation, they typically say they are using an app on their phone, which can be helpful. However, when I ask them if they are getting "good fertile mucus," I often get the response, "How would I know?" or "How would I check for that?"

This is important because if you aren't getting good cervical mucus at ovulation, it can impact whether the sperm even makes it into the uterus, let alone the fallopian tube where it would fertilize an egg.

You need to see the slippery-clear or very stretchy type of cervical mucus in a good enough supply so that alkaline sperm have the buffer that good cervical mucus provides so an acidic vaginal environment doesn't kill them off.

CERVICAL MUCUS TYPES & CHARACTERISTICS

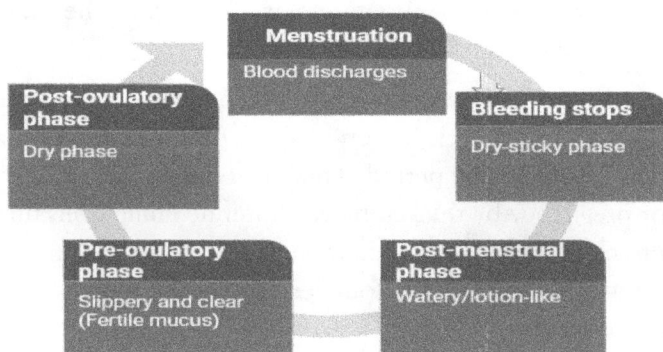

There are five different phases in the menstrual cycle. Each phase has its importance with cervical fluids or lack thereof and how it relates to the menstrual cycle regulation and fertility.

Locating Different Phases of Cervical Mucus

There should only be bleeding during your period, so you will not look for cervical mucus (CM) until you've stopped spotting.

What is considered normal with cervical mucus at each stage in the cycle:

- Menstruation: Blood discharges so that the uterus can be cleared and a new endometrial lining can form (three to seven days are typical, but some are longer). There is no cervical mucus during your period.

- Bleeding stops: The dry phase lasts for about a day or two after the bleeding has stopped, and normally, you won't notice any cervical mucus.

- Postmenstrual: After the dry phase, your discharge should become watery or lotion-like.

- Preovulatory: Usually around days 11–15, your discharge should become lotion-like, then turn a more slippery consistency as ovulation approaches. It could occur earlier or later, depending on your cycle length and how soon progesterone increases. Some women will experience the cervical mucus stretching about an inch between the first finger and thumb.

  During this phase, a mature egg (ovum) is released from one of the ovaries. After it's released, the egg moves down the fallopian tube and stays there for 12 to 24 hours, where it can be fertilized. It generally occurs about two weeks before the start of the menstrual period.

- Postovulatory: The luteal phase happens in the second part of your menstrual cycle, around day 15 of a 28-day cycle, and ends when you get your period. The luteal phase prepares your uterus for pregnancy by thickening your uterine lining even further so it is thick enough for implantation to take place, making it more receptive for the embryo. Your cervical mucus should be dry during this phase.

A good supply of progesterone during the luteal phase is important, as an insufficiency can affect becoming and staying pregnant. If you note discharge through this phase to when your period starts, you may need to make changes in your diet and lifestyle, as continuous discharge shouldn't last through the whole luteal phase.

These phases are equally important! Each depends on specific hormones being produced and utilized to support each phase of the cycle. If any of the hormones are not there to do their job, it can disrupt the cycle and any success with implantation and pregnancy.

The shorter the cycle, the earlier ovulation may occur, whereas the opposite is true with longer cycles. For example, a 36-day cycle would mean ovulation could occur as late as Day 24, maybe even Day 26, if the luteal phase is not as strong with the hormones that should be signaling then.

After ovulation, cells in the ovary release progesterone and a small amount of estrogen, which causes the uterus lining to thicken in preparation for pregnancy.

Luteal Phase Defect (LPD) occurs when a woman's ovaries don't release enough progesterone or the uterus lining doesn't respond to progesterone. It's also evident when charting shows the temperatures do not remain elevated after ovulation.

METHODS OF TRACKING OVULATION

Throughout your cycle, luteinizing hormone (LH) levels fluctuate and "surge" or significantly increase approximately 24 to 36 hours before ovulation. This surge stimulates the release of an egg from the ovary follicle, allowing it to travel down the fallopian tube.

Tracking your ovulation by combining old methods with newer technology will give you more certainty about when to expect ovulation to occur. Becoming familiar with your cervical fluid changes and other signs indicating ovulation is close is important. We'll get into detail on what will help you have better ovulations and a smoother premenstrual time, ideally with no hormonal symptoms.

Looking at BBT charting can help you understand what is "normal" and clarify when you should be most fertile. This should be done in addition to using an OPK, as some unexpected hormonal shifts can occur throughout your cycle that could cause a false positive signal.

OPKs will show you luteinizing hormone surges. Keep in mind that if you only use an OPK reading, you may not be able to tell whether it's your ovulation or a "false ovulation surge."

Women can experience false surges of luteinizing hormone when using an OPK. This can lead to false-positive or false-negative results, impacting the accuracy of the test in predicting ovulation. Conditions such as polycystic ovarian syndrome (PCOS) can cause irregularities in LH levels, making traditional OPKs unreliable.

Additionally, some women may experience mini-LH peaks throughout their cycle before the real LH surge that leads to ovulation, leading to false-positive results, so it's important to note that OPKs cannot confirm whether ovulation occurs.

Therefore, other methods, such as tracking basal body temperature and cervical mucus, may be used with OPKs to predict ovulation more accurately.

SOME OVULATION PREDICTOR KITS HAVE FLAWS

An unfortunate problem with most ovulation predictor kits is that while the test can estimate the time that ovulation should take place, it cannot determine if ovulation has occurred.

In some cases of infertility, such as LUFS (luteinized unruptured follicle syndrome), a woman experiences a surge in LH, but an egg is never released. So, even though the OPK is "positive," indicating the rise in LH (that occurs before ovulation) has occurred, the woman still doesn't conceive because she didn't ovulate (more about LUFS later).

If a woman has PCOS, the ovulation kits are not useful in predicting fertility. This is because PCOS can cause several spikes in LH levels, even without ovulation, so the ovulation test kit can show confusing results.

Likewise, women who experience a decline in fertility as they get closer to menopause may experience higher levels of luteinizing hormone, which can result in the ovulation prediction test giving false positive results for ovulation.

If a woman's LH surges last less than 10 hours and only uses the OPK once daily, she might miss her LH surge depending on when she tested.

OPKs can also have inaccuracies if a woman undergoing hormone therapy is pregnant, postpartum, or breastfeeding.

OPKs to try with more accurate outcomes: Clearblue Fertility Monitor or Ova Cure Fertility Monitor. Neither are without error nor are they 100% accurate. Charting your key fertility signs is still one of the best ways to boost your fertility and maximize your chances of conception!

BASAL BODY TEMPERATURE (BBT) CHARTING

I recommend that women also learn to use the basal body temperature method with a good working thermometer as another ovulation predictor. Take the time to get to know your cervix's location and the different secretions that come from there, depending on your cycle phase.

You may consider it "old school" these days to check using BBT, but if your OPK is giving you some hormonal inaccuracies, your body will let you know how close you are to ovulating by cervical location and the type of cervical mucus secreted.

The following link will walk you through the best way to check your cervix to know the different types of discharge occurring depending on where you are in your cycle: wikihow.com/Feel-Your-Cervix.

- Taking your BBT every morning at the same time consistently, without getting up first to use the restroom, is more accurate. Try to do this for at least three months to see your pattern. This can reveal what type of patterns are presenting themselves and also show the positive changes made by following a good fertility program.

- You'll also see when a better chance at conception can occur when a good graph is present.

- If you're not noting any good fertile cervical mucus at mid-cycle, you'll learn how to make it ideal here.

- If you haven't charted before, please refer to the Basal Body Temperature chart link in the Resources section.

Normally, at ovulation, the chart will show a dip in temperature followed by a .6 to 1 degree rise in temperature. A good ovulation will often maintain that post-ovulatory high for at least two to three days before it dips in temperature.

It's best to see only a few small dips (.2 to .3) occur in the luteal phase, as it usually indicates that progesterone is stable and doing its job to help implantation occur and stay in place.

THINGS TO CHECK TO BE SURE OF GOOD OVULATIONS

If you do have a 26- to 32-day cycle, the following is what you'll want to check to be more certain that ovulation is occurring.

1. Clear fallopian tubes—the only way you'll know that at least one or both ovaries are clear is if you conceived not long ago, or you've had a hysterosalpingogram (HSG) that shows they're clear.

2. Are you getting good cervical mucus mid-cycle (clear, slippery, or stretchy)? How can you check this? You can either determine this

when you wipe after urination and notice a slicker feeling when wiping or by inserting a finger into the vagina, up to the cervix, and testing the quality that way.

By stretchy, I mean that when you put the cervical mucus between your index finger and thumb, you can pull them apart slowly. If the mucus breaks apart with barely any separation, it's not quite fertile yet, but if it stretches to an inch apart or more, it would likely be good fertile mucus.

3. Use a BBT chart or an app on your phone to know the time of possible ovulation. It is seen as a small dip in the temperature followed by a surge of at least a .6 to 1.0-degree rise in temperature.

4. Luteal temperatures should stay elevated at least three days post-rise (preferably above 98.2 degrees) before making a small dip.

5. If the luteal phase is less than 10 days, test your progesterone levels. Typically, progesterone levels are at their "peak" at the mid-luteal phase, so if you have menses every 26 days (with ovulation predicted on day 13), then you should test your progesterone on cycle days 18 or 19 when it should be at its peak in the luteal phase.

If you know your peak time and it's regular, plan to have sex daily, unless hubby's sperm is low, then go for every other day from around day 10 of your cycle to day 16 if your cycle is around 28 days. If your cycle is longer than that, plan to continue to day 18 (32-day cycle) and up to days 22-24 (with a 36-day cycle).

You'll want to rule out any potential issues via testing that could be affecting ovulation:

- Ultrasound/sonogram (checking uterus, fallopian tubes, and ovaries)
- HSG (checks for clear tubes)
- STDs such as gonorrhea and syphilis, HIV/AIDS, and Hepatitis B
- HPV or other strains of herpes virus, chlamydia, yeast/candida, bacterial vaginosis, or other infections (pap smear and blood test, urinalysis)
- Laparoscopy (usually used when endometriosis symptoms are present or if there could be adhesions causing painful periods or infertility)

IS LUFS AFFECTING YOUR FERTILITY?

Some issues can get in the way of ovulation that testing may reveal. I'm referring to luteinizing unruptured follicle syndrome (LUFS).

In normal menstrual cycles, the ruptured follicle becomes a corpus luteum, which releases progesterone and stimulates the lining of the uterus to build up. However, with LUFS, even though the follicle never ruptures, it still releases progesterone.

From the outside, your cycle will look completely normal: you'll still get a regular period each month, and you'll still get positive results with the temperature method or ovulation sticks. The only way to detect LUFS is via ultrasound. It's also called "trapped egg syndrome."

Women with "unexplained" infertility may experience this phenomenon more often than fertile women, but the true incidence of this problem in both the fertile and infertile populations is unknown. LUFS is considered a "silent" problem because it often does not show symptoms and is not easily detected.[11]

Often, there is no apparent cause. However, long-term use of anti-inflammatory drugs (NSAIDs) and even some anti-inflammatory supplements may prevent the follicle from bursting free of the ovaries, leading to LUFS.

If you're taking anti-inflammatory drugs for chronic conditions like autoimmune diseases, arthritis, or endometriosis, you may want to talk to your doctor about possible impacts on your fertility or avoid them around the time that you should be ovulating.

These are some risk factors for LUFS:

- Unexplained infertility
- Endometriosis
- Pelvic adhesions
- Blocked fallopian tubes
- Use of nonsteroidal anti-inflammatory drugs (NSAIDs) such as aspirin, ibuprofen, and naproxen sodium.

LUFS doesn't necessarily happen every cycle, so while it may be a handicap to getting pregnant, it may just take slightly longer due to multiple cycles.

ACTION PLAN

1. Get a journal where you can track your periods and list the answers to all the questions about your cycle there. Doing this now will be an excellent way to track your changes.

2. Go through all the symptoms listed at the beginning of this chapter and note symptoms you have with your cycles and if there have been any changes of getting heavier, lighter, or irregular.

3. If you note these symptoms, you'll more clearly see which pattern(s) fit you best. We'll cover patterns commonly seen with the cycles and what to do to help regulate them. Track your cycle on an app or print out a paper BBT chart (see bonuses).

If you've already been doing this, great! If not, this is a good time to start. You can also list the OPK results to compare when they say you're ovulating and what you find with your temperatures and cervical mucus.

See if you get good cervical mucus after completing your menses. Note if there's a lot (more than a tsp) or if it's hard to notice any by inserting a finger toward your cervix to check. You may be able to see that there's fertile mucus by wiping after urination. Usually, wiping will feel very slick or slippery if you're closer to ovulation.

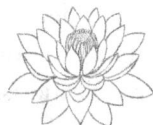

TESTING, *Testing,*
1, 2, 3

"There is purpose in your season of waiting."

—MEGAN SMALLEY

As of April 2022, in the United States, among heterosexual women aged 15 to 49 years with no prior births, about 1 in 5 (19%) are unable to get pregnant after one year of trying (infertility). Also, about 1 in 4 (26%) women in this group have difficulty getting pregnant or carrying a pregnancy to term. Male infertility plays a role in a couple's difficulty conceiving in anywhere from 35% to 50% of cases.

This isn't just occurring in the U.S. but also around the world, with 186 million individuals and 48 million couples having fertility issues.[12]

The decline in U.S. fertility has been driven primarily by a trend among young adults to postpone having children. Forty years ago, birth rates among women in their 20s were significantly higher than those in their 30s, but today, women are waiting until their 30s and sometimes early 40s to conceive.[13]

Some statistics say that the decline is from the rise in sexually transmitted diseases each year. In contrast, others say that times of economic stress can also play a role in infertility. I think that both can play a part.

Financial challenges can be an issue, especially if you need to seek out a fertility clinic, can't afford daycare, or there are no family or friends nearby to help with a newborn.

There are also more health-related issues due to toxins and heavy metals in the environment, diets high in processed foods, high sugar and carbohydrate concentration, high alcohol intake, and the depletion of nutrients in the soil where our fruits and vegetables grow.

Also, there are more drugs given for depression, anxiety, acid reflux, asthma, and allergies, not to mention high blood pressure and diabetes. If you or your partner are taking any medications, I would ask your pharmacist about the impact on fertility. Some of these medications are necessary and lifesaving, but check them to see how they could impact fertility.

In this chapter, we'll go over the different types of tests, including blood labs and other methods of testing that can give you and your partner the answers you need so you'll know what may be impacting your fertility and how to optimize it.

Earlier in the book, I shared the list of what is commonly tested and the observations made in a more general fertility assessment with a doctor, which is not enough in many cases, but they can be a good starting point.

We'll look at all the tests that can give answers to the diagnosis of "unexplained infertility." Most fertility cases have an explanation; they just require more tests. However, testing can get expensive, especially if you look into areas such as genetics, autoimmune factors, leaky gut, IBS, mold issues, systemic inflammation, and Lyme disease.

WHAT SHOULD BE TESTED

Hormones

Balance is important between estrogen and progesterone, as too much estrogen messes with the balance of progesterone. Balance is everything! Whether it's in your gut or "microbiome," every area must maintain a state of homeostasis to work most effectively.

If your total estrogens (estrone, estradiol, estriol, and estetrol) are too high, they will throw off your progesterone levels, typically lowering them.

Estradiol is the predominant estrogen during reproductive years. You need estrogen to nourish follicles and to grow a good endometrium for implantation.

If estrogens remain high and your progesterone doesn't rise in the luteal phase and stay elevated, it can impact implantation and the ability to hold a pregnancy.

These are the normal range numbers you want to see on your hormone labs:

Estradiol

- In adult males: 14 to 55 pg/mL
- In adult females estradiol fluctuates throughout the cycle:
    - ◦ Follicular phase (day 5)—19 to 140 pg/ml
    - ◦ Just before ovulation—110 to 410 pg/mL
    - ◦ Luteal phase—19 to 160 pg/ml
    - ◦ After menopause—less than 35 pg/ml[14]

Total Estrogens

- Follicular Phase (1-12 days)—90 to 590 pg/mL
- Luteal Phase—130 to 460 pg/mL

Progesterone

- During ovulation—1.8 to 24 ng/mL (best taken on day 21 of a 28-day cycle)

FSH (follicle-stimulating hormone)

- 3.85 to 8.78 IU/mL (should be taken on day 3 of menses)

AMH (anti-Mullerian hormone)

- 2 to 6.8 ng/ml (can be taken at any time of your cycle)

LH (luteinizing hormone)

- At the beginning of the cycle: 1.68 to 15 IU/L
- Mid-cycle peak, around the middle of the cycle: 21.9 to 56.6 IU/L
- Luteal phase, which is the end of the cycle: 0.61 to 16.3 IU/L

Prolactin

- Should be less than 25 ng/mL (high levels can impact fertility)

DHEA-S (stress hormone, needed for egg quality)

- For women, an ideal blood level is 275 ug/dL to 400 ug/dL
- For men, it's 350 ug/dL to 500 ug/dL

Testosterone (needed for egg in a balanced amount)

- For women ages 19 and up, normal testosterone levels range from 15 to 70 ng/dL.

Androstenedione

- 0.7 to 3.1 ng/mL

Blood Labs

- Complete blood count w/differential
- B12/folate (to check for anemia)
- Iron level (serum iron, TIBC, ferritin, iron saturation)

Anemia

Anemia, having insufficient levels of iron in the body, is important to remedy when trying to conceive. You need a good blood supply since so much goes to the developing embryo, and you want to have enough for both of you to thrive.

The two common types of anemia are iron deficiency and B12/folate deficiency (pernicious anemia). A low level of vitamin B12 in the blood indicates pernicious anemia. However, a false normal or high value of vitamin B12 in the blood may occur if antibodies interfere with the test.

Anemia can significantly impact female fertility, leading to irregular periods, difficulty ovulating, and other reproductive issues, so it is essential to address this before conception. If you have anemia, your body focuses on sending oxygen to vital organs like the brain and heart, leaving less oxygen for other body parts, including the reproductive system. This can increase the risk of miscarriage or premature birth if a woman does become pregnant.

High levels of homocysteine and methylmalonic acid (urine test) in your body can indicate pernicious anemia.

Other important blood tests to have checked (these can be part of a comprehensive panel):

- Fasting glucose, fasting insulin, and HA1C (Check for insulin resistance and prediabetes as imbalanced sugar levels can impact reproductive hormones negatively.)

- Homocysteine: If the levels of this amino acid are high, it usually indicates a deficiency in B6, folate, and B12. These nutrients are necessary in each body cell to fuel the mitochondria. (Mitochondria are like the power plants of the cell.) A high homocysteine level can contribute to arterial damage and blood clots in your blood vessels.

- C-reactive protein (an inflammatory marker): This protein is vital in the defense against inflammation and is made in the liver. When there is infection and trauma in the body, CRP levels can become high, but small increases above the baseline have been found to predict low-grade inflammation. Conditions characterized by low-grade inflammation are obesity, depression, or chronic pain.

  Chronic inflammation, which can be determined by looking at serum high-sensitivity C-reactive protein levels, has been linked with reduced rates of fertility, recurring miscarriages, and IVF failures.[15]

- Thyroid levels: TSH, free T3 & T4, TPO, TGA (It's important to have a stable level of thyroid hormones as estrogen rises.) Excessive estrogens can lower thyroid hormone levels.

- Liver markers: AST, ALT, GGT (Since your liver converts hormones into an absorbable and safe hormone, it needs to work well.)

- Fibrinogen: It helps to determine whether you have a bleeding or blood clotting disorder. Fibrinogen is an essential protein made by your liver. Excess fibrinogen can lead to clots.

- Vitamin D3: It's essential to have a more than adequate supply for hormone production and bone health, as the first trimester requires a lot in the "building and growth" stage. It also strengthens the nervous and immune systems.

- Lipids and triglycerides: Cholesterol, though often given a bad reputation, is important in the production of hormones, but too high a level of low-density lipoprotein (LDL), as well as elevated triglycerides, can point toward inflammation and possible early fatty liver disease. Fatty liver is something to watch for when liver enzymes are either high or on the high end of the normal range.

This information is important because you need to investigate anything depleting the substances that make important hormones for reproduction. If LDL markers, triglycerides, and liver markers are not elevated, then taking medication for cholesterol that is between 200 to 240 may not be necessary.

- Serum Zinc: Many studies have shown that zinc levels in the seminal plasma are positively associated with male fertility and that zinc supplementation may significantly increase semen volume, sperm motility, and the percentage of normal sperm morphology.[16]

Zinc is critical in processes that lead to creating eggs in the ovaries and supporting fertility and pregnancy.[17]

Regarding heart disease or concerns of systemic inflammation affecting heart health and the cardiovascular system, your doctor should check the following inflammatory markers: CRP, fibrinogen, LDL, triglycerides, platelets, ESR, and ferritin.

If they are elevated, taking anti-inflammatory supplements to lower inflammation and changing diet and lifestyle will be very important, and medication may be needed if levels are too high. Too much inflammation in the body can impair the reproductive process.

Inflammation is a normal bodily process in response to infection or injury; however, if prolonged inflammation persists, it can negatively impact fertility, your menstrual cycle, and implantation. It can also lead to endometriosis or result in recurrent miscarriage.

HSG

Hysterosalpingography, or HSG, is an X-ray test to outline the internal shape of the uterus and show whether the fallopian tubes are blocked. In HSG, a thin tube is threaded through the vagina and cervix, and a substance known as contrast material is injected into the uterus.

This is an important test because if there are any blockages from scar tissue (past infection) or endometrial tissue, an ectopic pregnancy could occur. Sometimes, simply clearing the tubes with this procedure can help with conception.

There are times when false blockages can be diagnosed, as the procedure can be uncomfortable and cause spasms in the tubes, which could keep the contrast from moving through them. This can sometimes happen, but more often, it is a very helpful diagnostic.

This can also be an opportunity to rule out cervical stenosis, which is a narrowing of the cervical canal. There's no test for this currently, but a HSG test, where the cannula has to pass through the cervix, can reveal tension or a narrowed passage. The concern with having narrowing of the cervix (stenosis) is that it could cause blood flow to go in the reverse direction (retrograde menstruation).

Because cervical stenosis is difficult to suspect and diagnose, many cases may go unnoticed until and unless the cervix is evaluated. This evaluation becomes more pressing in cases with certain risk factors such as endometriosis, polyps, and myomas. A prior history of endometriosis, reproductive tract surgery, polyps, and pelvic inflammatory disease were significantly associated with cervical stenosis.

Cervical dilation is the method used in Western medical treatment, but vaginal steaming may also be of benefit to help soften tissue that is causing constriction there.

Ultrasound/Sonogram

Your first transvaginal ultrasound is normally done on the first day of your period; this is known as your baseline ultrasound. The purpose is to check that there are no unusual cysts on the ovaries. Different types of ultrasounds can scan for infertility, including a baseline check or screening ultrasounds done to assess the pelvic anatomy of the uterus, including uterine lining and bilateral ovaries.

All abnormal findings are measured and characterized, such as fibroids, uterine malformations, hydrosalpinxes, and ovarian cysts, if any are present. It is important to know if you aren't aware of these already. Each can affect your ability to conceive, but knowledge of them will help you decide how to remedy them, if possible.

Pap Smear

Besides being used as a screening to detect cervical cancer or cell changes that may lead to cervical cancer, a Pap smear may also help find other conditions, such as infections or inflammation. Infections can harm the cervical environment if you are trying to conceive. It is also important to rule out human papillomavirus (HPV) before conception.

Candida

Candida overgrowth doesn't kill sperm, but because the infection changes the consistency of the cervical mucus, it may make it more difficult for the sperm to reach the cervical opening. Inflammation from the body trying to fight the infection is hostile to sperm. It is important to take steps to take care of this with dietary changes, probiotics, and herbs to rebalance the vagina. Also, your partner can keep giving it back to you if he isn't treated as well. If you only take over-the-counter medications and don't make diet and lifestyle changes, it can keep reoccurring.

Bacterial Vaginosis (BV) or Other Infections

Bacterial vaginosis (BV) and other infections can decrease fertility in several ways. Infections increase inflammation and immune system activity, which creates a toxic environment for reproduction. They can also cause damage to sperm and vaginal cells, which interferes with the production of healthy cervical mucus during ovulation.

Keeping your gut and vaginal microbiome in balance is very important in avoiding occurrences of BV. Wearing 100% cotton underwear will help lessen excess moisture and help the area have better air circulation.

If you swim or work out, remove any wet or damp clothing as soon as possible. Keeping underwear or bathing suit bottoms on too long will keep dampness locked next to the vulva and increase the chances of fungal infections and bacteria.

STDs: Chlamydia, Hepatitis C, Syphilis, Gonorrhea

Chlamydia is an STD that can silently cause problems for those wishing to conceive naturally. If not detected, this type of infection can infect the fallopian tubes, leading to scarring, narrowing, and less room for a fertilized egg (embryo) to get to the uterus to implant into the lining.

If you are going to a fertility specialist, they will perform this routine test, but if you aren't going to one yet, have your OB/GYN do this for you. It's normally done with your annual Pap smear, but I would do it as soon as possible to rule it out.

PELVIC HEALTH AND BLOOD CIRCULATION—WHAT IS IDEAL?

Your lower abdomen and reproductive organs need a good supply of nutrients and hormone signaling from the brain (hypothalamus, pituitary). Inadequate blood flow through the uterine artery will impact the embryo's growth. How would you know if this was happening?

A method I recommend is to check your skin temperature by touch. If your hands are typically cold or too hot, you'll want to pick up an infrared thermometer to measure the temperature of your lower abdomen just above the pubic bone. It should measure between 97.7 and 99 degrees. If the number is below that, then using topical warming techniques, massage, and deep abdominal breathing is important, as well as warming up your diet and drink options.

Topical Warming Options

- A hot water bottle or castor oil pack is used with a hot water bottle over your lower abdomen.

- Abdominal massage: See below for fallopian tube opening massage.

- Deep abdominal breathing: Make sure you take time every day to take breaths that are deep enough to cause your lower abdomen to rise. If you're not used to this, practice deep breathing with your hands over the area to feel it rise. Do this until you're used to breathing this way.

- Warming foods: Avoid raw fruits and vegetables, especially in winter. Adding more cooked, sautéed, or baked vegetables and meat dishes is also better for your digestion.

- Drinks: Avoid iced beverages or cold drinks; instead, drink warm or hot teas and room temperature or filtered warm water. To add warmth to your body, try drinking hot teas that include ginger or cinnamon, or a decaf chai tea, which can be a good option.

I love to make my own decaf chai tea in the fall and winter months. It's great before bed and can warm you from head to toe, but it shouldn't affect your sleep.

Decaf Chai Tea Recipe:

Put 2 cups of pure filtered water in a saucepan. Add:

- ° 6-8 cardamom pods
- ° 2 cinnamon sticks
- ° 6 cloves
- ° 1 knuckle-size piece of fresh ginger root
- ° 6-7 black pepper pods

Let them come to a slow boil for 10-15 minutes, then strain into a cup, add a little honey or stevia, and a nut milk of choice, and enjoy!

FALLOPIAN TUBE OPENING MASSAGE

Another type of therapy to encourage movement and circulation of fluids through the fallopian tubes is to massage along the lower abdomen, just above the pubic bone, toward the hips. (Only practice this next technique between menses and before ovulation when you are TTC.)

1. From the uterus (on the midline just above the pubic bone), you'll want to massage in a small circular clockwise motion with the pads of your fingers. Start in the middle, then move toward your hip and back. (Go as far as the hip bone when moving outward with your massage.)

2. With your fingertips, note areas of tension and congestion and apply deeper pressure, holding at the tighter regions. (This may be uncomfortable.) Make sure that you are breathing out when you press into areas of discomfort and then inhale as you ease off.

3. End the massage by using a pumping motion with the heel of the hand when you are in front of the hip bone area to encourage blood flow movement through the area.

ACTION PLAN

1. Set up appointments for you and your partner to have comprehensive blood, hormone, and STDs tested.

2. Schedule a Pap smear, HSG, and sonogram to determine if there are any issues.

3. If your hands are warm but your abdomen feels cool, spend time before bed with a hot water bottle and warm, non-caffeinated tea to help circulation.

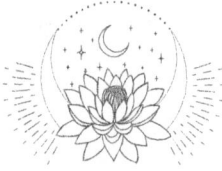

ISSUES THAT MAY IMPACT
Fertility

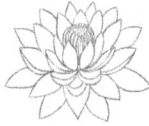

LOCAL OR SYSTEMIC
Inflammation AND *Autoimmunity*

"Never let the odds keep you from
doing what you know in your
heart you were meant to do."

—ANONYMOUS

A high percentage of gynecologic diseases, especially for women in their reproductive years, are caused by inflammation. Inflammation is a primary method by which we respond to infection, irritation, or injury. Your body's warning signal tells your immune system to check out what's happening and fix it.

Inflammation signals your immune system to pay attention to specific tissues in the body. It can be acute, like when you get a cut or a cold. When something is wrong, the immune system will do what it can to remove the offender, but if inflammation sticks around for too long because of issues such as a poor diet or chronic stress, it can overwhelm your body.

For women, inflammation can affect ovulation and hormone production and be associated with endometriosis.[18] Although the quality of the embryo mainly determines whether the egg is implanted successfully, other common medical conditions can also decrease implantation, including endometriosis and polycystic ovary syndrome, as well as uterine polyps and fibroids.

Inflammation has a significant role in gynecology and infertility, affecting the ovaries and uterus as well as the embryo and implantation.

SYMPTOMS OF INFLAMMATION

Normally, pain is a symptom of inflammation, but chlamydia, for example, which is a cause of infertility, is often asymptomatic. In this case, pain may not be a symptom unless it develops into pelvic inflammatory disease (PID).

Endometriosis also causes inflammation and will have pain symptoms in about 97% of cases.

You can test to tell you whether there is localized pelvic inflammation. If you're not having painful menses but are uncertain if inflammation is an issue, blood tests can help to understand what may be occurring.

Autoimmune diseases, sometimes called inflammatory diseases, are also caused by an overactive immune system that is out of balance. This is important if there's a history of miscarriages or years of issues with trying to conceive.

A fertility specialist should be able to do autoimmune testing for you if your primary doctor can't. Testing the following key markers for inflammation would be helpful in this case:

- Antinuclear antibodies (ANAs)
- Comprehensive NK cell assay
- TNF-alpha
- C-reactive protein (CRP)
- Antiphospholipid antibodies (APA)

AUTOIMMUNITY

Wikipedia describes autoimmunity as "the system of immune responses of an organism against its healthy cells and tissues. Any disease resulting from this immune response is termed an autoimmune disease."[19]

Chronic inflammation involves constant immune activation; the body floods with inflammatory cytokines. This occurs when the immune system faces an overabundance of triggers, including environmental toxins, food sensitivities, and chronic stress.

Immune problems associated with infertility and implantation failure tend to be more severe than those associated with miscarriage. Alan E. Beer, M.D., an expert on autoimmune infertility and author of *Is Your Body Baby-Friendly*, recommends that a woman has an endometrial biopsy on cycle day 26 to detect the presence of any harmful immune cells in her uterus.[20]

Treatment to regulate an overactive immune system can help if done faithfully for at least three months before trying to conceive. Often, supplements that reduce inflammation and oxidative damage and support the immune system can help achieve this. Many of the supplements listed in this book are for those very things!

An overactive immune system can cause damage to the placenta and cause a miscarriage. It can also damage the embryo and lead to implantation failure. Some autoimmune conditions can be linked to repeated miscarriages.

There are over a hundred different autoimmune diseases, but here are some common health issues that aren't always understood to be autoimmune diseases: celiac, Crohn's, psoriasis, endometriosis, fibromyalgia, Graves' disease, Hashimoto's thyroiditis, interstitial cystitis, lupus, Lyme disease, Ménière's disease, peripheral neuropathy, rheumatoid arthritis, and type 1 diabetes.

Some of these autoimmune conditions can directly cause infertility, while others are more indirect. One autoimmune condition can lead to another condition that may impact fertility.[21]

Peripheral neuropathy is a good example of this. There is no evidence to suggest that peripheral neuropathy can directly cause infertility. However, neuropathy can cause sexual dysfunction in men, which can lead to infertility through erectile dysfunction, ejaculatory dysfunction, and semen abnormalities.

Additionally, diabetes, which is a common cause of peripheral neuropathy, can have a significant effect on male reproductive function, leading to semen abnormalities due to overt ejaculatory dysfunction.

Blood clotting factors can cause infertility in both females and males. Here are some ways it can impact females:

- Recurrent miscarriage: Excessive clotting is associated with recurrent miscarriage. Inherited thrombophilia, which is genetically caused blood clots, can also be a cause of miscarriage and unexplained infertility.

- Heavy menstrual bleeding: Bleeding and clotting disorders can cause heavy menstrual bleeding. This can lead to anemia, which can affect fertility.
- Complications of pregnancy: Bleeding and clotting disorders can cause complications during pregnancy, such as placental abruption, preterm labor, and pre-eclampsia.
- Decreased probability of pregnancy: An enhanced clot growth rate before in vitro fertilization decreases the probability of pregnancy.[22]

In men, hemophilia, which is caused by a deficiency of clotting factors, can lead to infertility. It is important to note that not all clotting disorders cause infertility, and not all cases of infertility are caused by clotting disorders.

It is important to know that your blood circulation flows smoothly throughout the reproductive area, especially the uterine artery, to the placenta that nourishes the baby once you're pregnant.

Also, for conception, you need your blood to be just the right consistency, not too thin or too thick, so your hormones and blood can get to the ovaries, vagina, and fallopian tubes.

It is normal for blood to clot when you get a cut, but if blood takes too long to clot and the blood is very thin and watery, there may be less clotting factor available.

The opposite is also true; if you have too much clotting factor, which can happen with some immune conditions, it can lead to a lack of blood circulation to the uterus and other reproductive organs where it's needed.

Your genetics determine your clotting factor. Prothrombin (how long it takes your blood to clot) and a platelet count are good to check (or a D-dimer test) if you are worried about spike proteins or have pain or clots with your menses.

If you have painful periods and larger clots, you will want to take anti-inflammatory supplements that help with blood viscosity. Some doctors will suggest taking baby aspirin, and this may be enough, but you may need something stronger, depending on your test results.

ACTION PLAN

1. List the positive changes you want to make (what you will give up that could improve your fertility outcome).

2. If you have suffered from recurrent miscarriages, have further testing done for antibodies or blood clotting issues. (Maybe too much or not enough clotting is the problem?)

3. Have your doctor test for MTHFR mutations, antiphospholipid antibody (APA), Factor V Leiden, and antinuclear antibodies (ANA), especially if you have been trying for over two years with the same partner and not conceiving or haven't been able to make it to full-term.

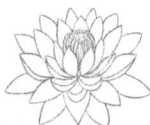

POLYCYSTIC OVARIAN SYNDROME (PCOS) AND OTHER *Ovarian Disorders*

"Never give up on a dream just because
of the time it will take to accomplish it."

—ANONYMOUS

After trying to conceive for three years without success, Tara started getting serious about tracking her ovulation. Fast forward four years, and she and her husband, Joe, still had not conceived.

Two years earlier, at age 34, Tara started delving deeper into why they weren't getting pregnant. She was having irregular cycles that would cause cramping and breast tenderness. After some testing, she found out that she had PCOS (polycystic ovary syndrome).

Her daily routine was anything but calm. She had a stressful job and found herself stress-eating, mainly anything sweet. With her work schedule, she rarely packed lunch and then would grab fast food on the way home, and she was about 20 pounds over her ideal weight. Her sleep was okay, but she'd find herself tired early in the day.

As you can imagine, when they came to see me, Tara and Joe were frustrated and scared that their dreams of having a baby would not happen. After an initial interview and exam, I recommended that Tara have some blood tests and an ultrasound to see what was going on inside, as well as determine why she was having pain in the upper right area of her abdomen.

We found out through a blood test and ultrasound that she had a fatty liver. Tara's symptoms with PCOS and fatty liver are common ones, and often, the stress, blood sugar highs and lows, and weight gain, as well as some inherent genetic factors, can lead to both of these diagnoses, besides viewing the ovaries for the high number of cysts found there.

To help with the fatty liver and to decrease inflammation, I worked with her on a program to change her eating habits and avoid all alcoholic beverages, processed foods, and starchy carbs. She started drinking more water and walking 20 minutes three to four times a week. Her liver needed to be cleared of excess sugars to begin working better to regulate hormones. I gave her an herbal formula and supplements to help her liver, regulate her blood sugar level and insulin resistance, and help her ovulate more consistently.

Joe had a reverse vasectomy that, unfortunately, wasn't working well via ejaculation, so any good viable sperm would have to be needle-extracted directly from the testes. Tara would have to go through in vitro fertilization to be able to use her husband's sperm.

Since they were going to do IVF, I was helping them prepare for this process. I wanted Tara to be on this protocol for at least three months before starting the medications for the egg retrieval process. We wanted to get her PCOS regulated as well as help her liver function optimally so that the first IVF round would have a better chance of working.

She also practiced daily guided meditation for fertility and to reduce stress. She found this helped her sleep and feel better at her job. Her diligence with the plan made a big difference, and Tara became pregnant.

IVFs don't always work the first time, as finding the correct dosage of medication and hormones for each individual is not easy. She was so grateful that she made the changes, as besides being so happy to conceive, she also lost 15 pounds before going through the in vitro procedure. Diet is so key!

Both chronic stress and sugary diets can lead to increased cortisol production and insulin resistance (where the cells are not getting the energy they need). This can cause problems with producing the necessary hormones to ovulate, including adequate levels of progesterone to help implant and hold a baby to term.

WHAT IS PCOS?

PCOS is a very common hormonal problem for women trying to conceive. The most common symptoms that women may experience are being unable to ovulate, having high levels of androgens like testosterone and luteinizing hormone but low levels of follicle-stimulating hormone, and having many small cysts on the ovaries. The number and size of the cysts can vary from the size of an almond to a grapefruit. Depending on their size, cysts can irritate the bladder and intestines. Pain and discomfort may also occur when cysts press against other tissues, burst, or increase in size.

PCOS can cause missed or irregular menstrual cycles, hair growth in undesired areas, acne on the face and/or back, infertility, and problems losing weight.[23] It can have similar symptoms to congenital adrenal hyperplasia. We'll look at the similarities between the two.

What can cause PCOS to occur? Here are some of the key factors:

- Hormonal imbalances with androgens, LH, FSH, progesterone, and estrogen
- Dietary factors
- Poor circulation of blood and lymph, which may cause pelvic congestion
- Liver dysfunction, which may cause improper synthesis and breakdown of hormones
- Infection from an abortion and IUD use
- Lack of exercise
- Constipation
- Insulin resistance, which may result in hormonal fluctuations and imbalances
- Appendicitis

TESTING FOR PCOS

Testing will involve checking for any hormone imbalances involved with menses and ovulation:

- A pituitary blockage or insufficiency in making follicle-stimulating hormone, and luteinizing hormone. Test these two.

- Thyroid imbalance: test TSH (thyroid-stimulating hormone), Thyroxine-T4, and T3.

- Chronic adrenal hyperplasia: test steroid panel and DHEA.

- Luteal Phase Defect: check to see if your temperatures stay elevated during the luteal phase on a BBT or have your progesterone tested at the peak of the luteal phase. Test progesterone midway between ovulation and your next period.

- Less cervical mucus due to insufficient estrogen: test a full hormone panel.

- Individual test: liver markers, lipid panel, fasting insulin, and HA1C should also be checked, as well as having an abdominal ultrasound done to view the ovaries.

- Having PCOS can increase the risk of miscarriage because of the higher blood levels of the luteinizing hormone often found in women with PCOS. Test luteinizing hormone levels.

INSULIN RESISTANCE AND PCOS

Insulin resistance is common with PCOS. If blood tests reveal high fasting glucose (blood sugar), your hemoglobin A1C (HA1C) is over 5.6, and fasting insulin is high, you may not get the necessary nutrients into your cells.

Insulin resistance is a condition where cells in the muscles, fat, and liver do not respond well to insulin and cannot easily take up glucose from the blood. Since balanced glucose levels are needed to give you and your cells energy, you may feel lethargic without enough glucose, like you need a nap, caffeine, or something sweet!

While genetics, aging, and ethnicity play roles in developing insulin sensitivity, the driving forces behind insulin resistance include excess body weight, too much belly fat, a lack of exercise, smoking, and even skimping on sleep.

Insulin is a hormone produced by the pancreas that helps glucose in the blood enter cells in the muscles, fat, and liver, where it is used for energy. When blood glucose levels rise after eating, the pancreas releases insulin into the blood, lowering blood glucose to keep it in the normal range.

If testing shows that you have insulin resistance, it's important to change your lifestyle for optimal fertility, as you'll need energy to get into the cells of the organs and glands that help reproduction.

Balancing blood sugar is very important, as the result of continuing to eat and drink processed and sugary foods can mean going from insulin-resistant to becoming diabetic. No one wants that to happen if it is avoidable.

Insulin resistance can impact fertility, particularly in women who are overweight or have PCOS. It can cause women to ovulate irregularly or not ovulate at all, which can result in infertility. Insulin resistance can also lead to hormonal imbalances, which can further contribute to reproductive problems. Treating insulin resistance can often make it possible for a woman to get pregnant, although sometimes additional fertility treatments are necessary. Patients with insulin resistance who are trying to get pregnant are often given metformin, an insulin-sensitizing drug.

Inflammation and insulin resistance can also have adverse effects on sperm quality in men. High insulin levels can cause inflammation and impact several hormones that relate to fertility, including testosterone, DHT, estrogen, and cholesterol. Therefore, reducing insulin resistance through lifestyle changes and medication can improve fertility outcomes for both men and women.[24]

CHANGING YOUR DIET

It's hard to do something about an issue if you're unaware it's happening in your body. The most important thing to remember with PCOS, if you know that you have it, is to make changes to your diet and lifestyle that help regulate insulin and balance blood sugar, as it can make a big difference. It will take some determination, but these changes may increase your fertility chances and overall health and longevity.

NONALCOHOLIC FATTY LIVER DISEASE (NAFLD)

NAFLD is a condition where fat builds up in the liver. It is closely linked to metabolic syndrome, a disorder characterized by the body's abnormal use and storage of energy. It is associated with an increased risk of heart disease, diabetes, and stroke.

NAFLD in infertile women with polycystic ovarian syndrome is a problem that needs to be checked with a blood test. The prevalence of NAFLD increases with age and is far more common among people who are obese and diabetic.[25] People with NAFLD and metabolic syndrome are usually insulin-resistant.

DIETARY CONSIDERATIONS FOR PCOS AND NAFLD

1. Avoid saturated fats. These interfere with hormones and liver function. Also, minimize red meats, high-fat dairy products, and fried foods.

2. Add essential fatty acids (EFAs), the beneficial fats in fish, nuts, and seeds.

3. Avoid alcohol, caffeinated coffee, tea, and processed and fried foods, as they may interfere with hormone function.

4. Magnesium is thought to regulate various hormones (e.g., androgens, LH, and FSH) and may also help reduce cramping and inflammation. Start with 300mg daily unless you have loose stools at that dose, then back to 200mg daily.

5. Avoid processed sugars, candy, sweets, aspartame, synthetic sweeteners, and high starch and carbohydrate foods.

WHAT IS ADRENAL HYPERPLASIA?

According to the Mayo Clinic, congenital adrenal hyperplasia (CAH) refers to a group of genetic disorders inherited from parents and present at birth that affect the adrenal glands, a pair of walnut-sized organs above the kidneys.

The adrenal glands produce essential hormones, including:

- Cortisol, which regulates the body's response to illness or stress.

- Mineralocorticoids, such as aldosterone, which regulate sodium and potassium levels.

- Androgens, such as testosterone, are male sex hormones required for growth and development in both males and females.

In people with CAH, a gene change (mutation) results in a lack of one of the enzymes needed to make these hormones. Although there is no cure, with proper treatment, most people who have CAH can lead full lives.

The two major types of congenital adrenal hyperplasia are classic CAH and nonclassic CAH.

Classic CAH

This form is rarer and more severe than nonclassic CAH. It is usually detected at birth or early infancy. Signs and symptoms may include:

- **Insufficient cortisol.** Classic CAH causes the body to produce an insufficient amount of cortisol. This can cause problems maintaining normal blood pressure, blood sugar, and energy levels and cause problems during physical stress such as illness.

- **Adrenal crisis.** People with classic CAH can be seriously affected by a lack of cortisol, aldosterone, or both. This is known as an adrenal crisis, and it can be life-threatening.

- **Atypical genitalia.** Female infants may have an atypical genitalia appearance, such as an enlarged clitoris that may resemble a penis and a partially closed labia resembling a scrotum. The urinary opening (urethra) and the vagina may be only one opening instead of two. The uterus, fallopian tubes, and ovaries usually develop normally. Male infants usually have typical-appearing genitals.

- **Excess androgen.** An excess of the male sex hormone androgen can result in short height and early puberty for both males and females. Pubic hair and other signs of puberty may appear at a very early age. Severe acne also may occur. Excess androgen hormones in females may result in facial hair, excessive body hair, and a deepening voice.

- **Altered growth.** Rapid growth may occur during childhood with an advanced bone age. The final height may be shorter than average.

- **Fertility issues.** Irregular menstrual periods, not having any at all, and infertility problems can occur in females. Fertility issues can sometimes occur in males with this.

Nonclassic CAH

Often there are no symptoms of nonclassic CAH when a baby is born. Some people with nonclassic CAH never have symptoms. The condition is not identified on routine infant blood screening and usually becomes evident in late childhood or early adulthood. Cortisol may be the only hormone that's deficient.

Females who have nonclassic CAH may have typical-appearing genitals at birth. Later in life, they may experience irregular menstrual periods, or not having any at all, and problems getting pregnant, along with masculine characteristics such as facial hair, excessive body hair, and a deepening voice.

In both females and males, signs of nonclassic CAH may also include early appearance of pubic hair and other signs of early puberty, severe acne, and rapid growth during childhood with an advanced bone age and shorter than expected final height.

Causes of CAH

The most common cause of CAH is the lack of the enzyme known as 21-hydroxylase. CAH may sometimes be called a 21-hydroxylase deficiency. Your body requires this enzyme to make proper amounts of hormones. There are other much rarer enzyme deficiencies that also cause CAH.

Children who have the condition have two parents who either have CAH themselves or who are carriers of the genetic change that causes the condition. This is known as the autosomal recessive inheritance pattern. Those found to be more susceptible are of Ashkenazi Jewish, Latino, Mediterranean, Yugoslav, or Yup'ik ancestry.

ACTION PLAN

1. If you have symptoms that were described in any of the conditions that have been discussed—PCOS, cysts, or symptoms of congenital adrenal hyperplasia—make an appointment with your OB/GYN to get tested.

2. If you've already been diagnosed with any of the reproductive issues mentioned, start tracking your symptoms each month as you start cleaning up your diet and lessening inflammatory foods, as well as regulating your blood sugar (this is important in all cases, but especially with PCOS).

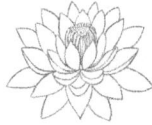

Endometriosis

"I am both powerful and desirable.
It is wonderful to be a woman.

I love myself, and I am fulfilled."

—LOUISE HAY

Endometriosis, a medical condition where the tissue that normally lines the inside of your uterus grows outside of it, can be a cause of infertility. It affects millions of women and is usually diagnosed between the ages of 30 and 40, but it can begin as early as the teenage years. Some have speculated that the uterus may be tilted or the opening of the cervix is too narrow, causing the menstrual blood to back up.

So how do you know if you have it? The most common symptoms of endometriosis are severe menstrual cramps (close to 97% of women with endometriosis do have menstrual pain). Women with endometriosis tend to have higher prostaglandin levels, which causes menstrual pain. Other common symptoms are irregular periods, back pain, infertility, pain during intercourse, pressure during bowel movements, feeling pressure on the bladder (so the need to urinate occurs more often), and chronic fatigue.

Although the cause is unknown, the major theory is that endometrial cells migrate during fetal development, or cells shed or expelled during menstruation travel upward through the fallopian tube(s).

Statistically, 25-50% of infertile patients have endometriosis.[26] Many women are undiagnosed, as their doctor hasn't realized all the different symptoms relating to endometriosis are ones that are present. Painful periods alone are just part of the "symptom picture."

Different depths can make a difference in whether it causes pain or not:

- Superficial: it sits on the surface of the membrane and seems to be more implicated in infertility.
- Deeper: penetrates a few millimeters into the membrane and the underlying tissues and causes pain.
- Around 40% of women diagnosed with this report no symptoms other than infertility.
- Common implantation sites can include the cervix, vaginal-rectal space, ovaries, fallopian tubes, colon, and bladder. (It has also been found in the abdominal wall, lungs, nose, and brain.)

Why is it more challenging to get pregnant with endometriosis?

- If scarring and adhesions are present, as with a severe case, it can block the egg's path to the uterus.
- It is possible that dysfunction in the ovaries, or the hormonal issues producing luteal phase defect, are causing problems that lead to endometriosis.

If you think of the proximity of the reproductive organs to the small and large intestines and bladder, it makes more sense how inflammation, or other problems in those tissues and organs, can affect reproduction:

- Prolapse of organs putting pressure on the reproductive system.
- Inflamed bowel or bladder.
- Adhesions in the abdomen irritate or affect the movement of the fallopian tubes or block blood flow to the uterus or ovaries.
- Dysfunction in your organs can lead to dysfunction in the uterus and vagina, cause menopausal disorders, and affect your period, fertility, and pregnancy.

Ask your doctor if you've not been diagnosed with endometriosis but have had painful periods or have tried to conceive without success and nothing else is blocking conception. More doctors are becoming aware of the ReceptivaDx way to test for the possibility of increased uterine inflammation or chances of endometriosis being present.

The ways that Western medicine may test for this is either by ultrasound (to identify cystic endometriosis), MRI, a pelvic exam (to locate painful areas), and the most helpful but invasive procedure is laparoscopy (which allows viewing the reproductive and local tissues for cysts, adhesions, or lesions of endometriosis as well as taking a biopsy for testing).[27]

Testing is essential; you may need to find an autoimmune fertility specialist to run specific labs to confirm how much inflammation is present. Knowing these results is particularly useful for early diagnosis of minimal to mild endometriosis, which can still affect fertility.

THE ACTION PLAN

- Follow an anti-inflammatory diet such as the anti-inflammatory Mediterranean Diet.
- Add omega-3s (in pill form) or eat more cod, salmon, trout, sardines, mussels, rapini, spinach, flax seeds, mangoes, lettuce, and kidney beans.
- Lessen omega-6 foods that create inflammation if they are already high in your diet. They are found in fried foods, rancid vegetable oils, and grain-fed beef (not grass-fed).
- Take antioxidants (see fertility supplement recommendations), and eat more organic, colorful vegetables and fruits daily.
- Yoni steam to help reduce/eliminate pain. Do these after menstrual bleeding is over to a couple of days before ovulation occurs. You can also do them before your period starts (but only on months when you're not TTC).

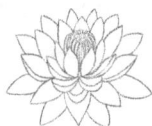

Fibroids, HYDROSALPINX, AND PID

"I am learning to trust the journey
even when I do not understand it."

—MILA BRON

I've treated many women in my clinic who were trying to conceive and found out that they had one or more fibroids in the uterus lining, muscle, or exterior. These fibroids can cause symptoms of heavy bleeding and pain with menses, but not always.

If you note some familiar symptoms after going through this chapter, I'd highly recommend getting an appointment with your OB/GYN as soon as possible.

FIBROIDS—COULD YOU HAVE MORE THAN ONE?

About 35% of all women over age 35 have fibroids, also known as myomas (most are benign and cause no symptoms). These fibroids may occur as an isolated growth, but there is likely to be more than one, and they will vary in size. Small ones are often symptomless, so you may not even know you have them until you start exploring reasons for infertility.

Excessive uterine bleeding is a common factor because the uterus lining expands from the pressure of the fibroid, causing an increased amount of tissue (maybe with larger-sized clots) with the menstrual blood. Large fibroids may press on the bladder and cause bladder symptoms such as urinary irritability and frequency or pain with urination. Fibroids can grow in three locations: on the inner wall, within the muscular wall, or on the outer wall of the uterus underneath the peritoneum.

How Can This Affect Fertility?

- Submucosal fibroids take up space in the endometrium and can prevent a fertilized egg from implanting.
- Fibroids located near the fallopian tubes can obstruct the passageway, making it impossible for the sperm to go up and eggs to come down.
- Fibroids compete for the blood supply of the uterus and often win out over a developing fetus.
- Cervical fibroids can distort the cervix and possibly affect the cervical mucus, interfering with the sperm.

What Is the Most Accurate Test for Fibroids?

One of the main tests to diagnose fibroids is an ultrasound scan. This painless scan uses a probe to produce high-frequency sound waves to create an image of the inside of your body. They can see where fibroids are located, what their size is, and where they are located in the uterus.

The treatments depend on the location and size of the fibroids. Many things can be done to shrink them if they are subserous (in the lining of the uterus), but it depends on the fibroid size. If they are small, then diet, lifestyle, castor oil packs, and specific herbs and supplements can help tremendously.

Larger fibroids, around four centimeters or more that are interstitial (in the muscle of the uterus), can impact implantation and might block the fallopian tubes, which can cause infertility.

It is hard to reduce large fibroids as cutting them out could cause damage to the uterus and its ability to hold a pregnancy. However, by implementing a plant-based diet to lower excess estrogens, stress, and inflammation, the fibroids might become small enough to be safely removed.

This is a diet I recommend that will give your body lots of nutrient-rich foods:

- Organic foods (the clean 15 foods are okay, but avoid the dirty dozen, which are the most heavily sprayed with pesticides!)[28]
- High-fiber foods, including cruciferous vegetables such as broccoli, cauliflower, cabbage, Brussels sprouts, and bok choy.
- Green leafy vegetables.
- Beta-carotene-rich foods (such as carrots and sweet potatoes).
- Foods high in iron (such as grass-fed beef and legumes), especially if there is heavy menstrual bleeding. Subserous fibroids tend to cause heavier menses.
- Flaxseeds contain phytoestrogen with fibroid healing properties.
- Buckwheat, quinoa, gluten-free oats (avoid gluten and dairy products).
- Fruits like apples and berries (blueberries, blackberries, raspberries, boysenberries).
- The Mediterranean diet is good as there are more vegetables and fish included.
- Avoid alcohol.
- Always buy organic, nonhormone, and not packaged in plastic if possible.

Since total estrogens are often high when fibroids are present, testing for total estrogen levels should be done.

The following supplements may help to regulate hormones and lower fibrin levels common in fibroid tumors:

1. Calcium D-Glucarate or D.I.M. to regulate estrogen levels.
2. Neprinol AFD or NATTO: to reduce fibrin levels (what fibroids are made of). Take this between meals on an empty stomach.

Other helpful things to add:

Yoni steaming (vaginal steams): between the end of your period (when not bleeding) and a few days before ovulation (if you are actively trying to conceive) on months when you aren't TTC, you can continue the yoni steams every couple of days up to your next cycle.

Castor oil packs are used over the liver area as often as possible. I'll have more information on that in the Resources section.

HYDROSALPINX

Another health risk to conception is hydrosalpinx. A hydrosalpinx is the blockage of a woman's fallopian tube caused by a fluid buildup and dilation of the tube at its end.

Most often, it occurs at the end of the tube next to the ovary, but it can also occur at the other end of the tube that attaches to the uterus.

When the fluid leaks down into the uterus, it can cause implantation issues. Often, the involved tube will need to be removed, as clamping the tube isn't always successful.

Hydrosalpinx is a serious threat to fertility. It not only renders the affected tube(s) ineffective, but it may also lessen the effectiveness of various infertility treatments, such as in vitro fertilization.

Hydrosalpinx also increases the likelihood of miscarriage. Fluid from a tube that spills into the uterus is considered to be toxic to embryos, so it decreases the chance of successful embryo implantation.

Pelvic pain and discharge that is discolored or sticky are possible symptoms.

What Can Cause Hydrosalpinx?

An untreated infection is the most common cause of hydrosalpinx. Harmful bacteria can damage your fallopian tubes and cause them to become inflamed.

This inflammation often happens at the part of your fallopian tube near your ovaries or your fimbriae. Your fimbriae are finger-like extensions that sweep an egg from your ovaries into your fallopian tubes.

As part of the healing process, your fimbriae may fuse, sealing your fallopian tubes. Fluid gets trapped inside your tubes, causing them to swell.

Hydrosalpinx can also be caused by previously untreated sexually transmitted infections (STIs) like chlamydia and gonorrhea; pelvic inflammatory disease, often resulting from untreated STIs; scar tissue left over from pelvic surgery, especially surgery on your fallopian tubes; tissue build-up from endometriosis; and some tumors.

Testing to Diagnose Hydrosalpinx

- Ultrasound.

- Hysterosalpingogram (HSG): This test is commonly checked for anyone who has been trying to conceive for a year or more to rule out blockage or absence of a tube.

- Laparoscopy.

- Laparotomy (open surgery).[29]

PELVIC INFLAMMATORY DISEASE

Pelvic inflammatory disease (PID) is another condition that can contribute to hydrosalpinx or scar tissue that hampers the movement of the fimbria at the end of the fallopian tubes. It is usually the result of a bacterial infection (often an STD) that enters the body via the vagina and cervix and, from there, spreads throughout the pelvic cavity.

If a woman suspects she has (or has had) PID, it's important to consult an MD for a diagnosis and possible antibiotic treatment if caught early on.

PID, if not detected early, can cause scar tissue that can lead to infertility by blocking areas of reproduction that are crucial for conception, such as:

- An ovary covered with adhesions blocking the mature egg from entering the pelvic cavity.

- The fallopian tube could be narrowed or even completely obstructed.

- The uterus could have scar tissue, causing a problem with implantation of a fertilized egg.

Techniques That May Open Blockages

Here are three specialty abdominal massages that may help soften and break up adhesions to improve fertility:

1. Chi Nei Tsang

2. Arvigo Mayan Massage

3. Clear Passage Therapy

Some practitioners of these styles of massage may have a clinic nearby. The cost of these can vary by location, and the Clear Passage is a bit expensive but could be covered by your insurance plan if pain is a common complaint. It's worth asking about.

ACTION PLAN

1. If you have symptoms that were described in any of the conditions in this chapter, make an appointment with your OB/GYN for an ultrasound and other diagnostics.

2. If you've already been diagnosed with any of the reproductive issues mentioned, start tracking your symptoms each month as you start cleaning up your diet and lessening inflammatory foods, doing castor oil packs, as well as vaginal steaming. Steams are best done after menstrual bleeding has stopped and continued every other day up to a day or two before ovulation.

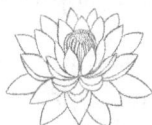

THYROID *Imbalances*

"Sometimes, struggles are exactly what we
need in our life. If we were to go through
our life without any obstacles, we would be
crippled. We would not be as strong as what
we could have been. Give every opportunity
a chance, leave no room for regrets."

—FRIEDRICH NIETZSCHE

At age 35, Connie and her husband had been trying to conceive for over a year. She'd had one miscarriage and was at her wit's end as to why she couldn't conceive and hold a pregnancy. She had a stressful job with symptoms of premenstrual breast tenderness, insomnia, lower back pain, and loose stools. She'd had her gallbladder removed many years ago due to obstruction (so she couldn't eat fatty foods).

She also complained to me that she had been getting headaches and having heart palpitations for several years. Before coming to see me, she and her husband tried IVF, as they wanted to have a baby as soon as possible and thought that this avenue would be their best option.

After talking at great length about their journey and reviewing their tests and findings from the fertility specialist, I sent her for more comprehensive lab testing. We discovered that her thyroid antibodies were high, indicating she had Hashimoto's thyroiditis, as well as some nutrient deficiencies.

Hashimoto's is an autoimmune disorder where the immune system attacks the thyroid's hormone-producing cells. If a woman doesn't know she has Hashimoto's when going through an IVF, the estrogens used to build the lining can further lower thyroid hormones that are necessary. If thyroid-stimulating hormone is the only thing tested for the health of the thyroid, it doesn't reveal Hashimoto's. The thyroid antibodies must be tested to know if this could be a factor. Many will have better results if they find a fertility clinic that specializes in autoimmunity, so they will know which drugs and hormones will be appropriate.

It took a year of acupuncture treatments to regulate her hormones, supplement nutrient deficiencies, and improve her diet to help her eggs get to a sound stage for a winning IVF treatment.

Their IVF procedure was successful, and they had a baby girl. In fact, a year later, they went through IVF again and added a son to their amazing family!

THYROID IMBALANCE

Did you know that 95% of those who have hypothyroidism may have Hashimoto's thyroiditis? As I mentioned at the beginning of the chapter, Hashimoto's is an autoimmune disease where your body makes antibodies that attack the cells in your thyroid gland. The symptoms may include an enlarged thyroid gland (goiter), fatigue, weight gain, muscle weakness, and more.

The increased occurrence of a high-normal level of TSH (thyroid stimulating hormone) and raised anti-thyroid peroxidase antibodies indicate a more frequent occurrence of lowered thyroid function in infertile women. This same study found that there is a greater tendency for thyroid disorder and elevated prolactin levels in infertile women than in fertile ones.[30] Not everyone with Hashimoto's disease will develop hypothyroidism, but it is the most common cause. If you have an underactive thyroid or too little thyroid hormone in your blood due to an issue like Hashimoto's, the body is unable to function normally.

Most patients with Hashimoto's and hypothyroidism will have acid reflux, nutrient deficiencies, anemia, leaky gut, food allergies, and adrenal insufficiency. Other symptoms that you might experience include impaired digestion/absorption, anxiety, chronic fatigue, and chemical/environmental allergies.[31]

Since Hashimoto's is an autoimmune condition that impairs absorption, the inflammation can negatively impact the thyroid gland, so it doesn't make enough of the hormones necessary to regulate the reproductive system.

If you already know that you have Hashimoto's, I suggest finding a naturopathic doctor in your area who can prescribe a gluten-free thyroid medication. Make sure the focus is on bringing down antibodies as quickly as possible. Diet and lifestyle are also essential.

If you are uncertain if you have a hypothyroid problem, it is good to have testing done, including a full thyroid panel with TPO and TgA included. Many doctors only test for thyroid-stimulating hormone (TSH), and that is not enough to rule out Hashimoto's.

Using the autoimmune Paleo diet and seeing your doctor for testing are good starting points. If they refuse to do a full thyroid panel, find a different doctor. I do these tests for my patients as you need to know what changes to make in your diet, lifestyle, and supplementation.

Sometimes, miscarriage can also happen when important thyroid hormones such as T4 and/or T3 are low. If there are problems with digestion and assimilation of nutrients, then the T4 may have problems converting to T3, which is the active form that fuels your metabolism and more. That is why it's important to not only have TSH measured but also the whole panel.

If total estrogen levels tend to run high in your body due to higher fatty food intake, an endocrine-disrupting environment that is converting to estrogen, and more, it can reduce your thyroid's ability to work as well. Estrogen dominance (higher levels than progesterone levels) has been found to lower T4/T3 levels. That is why many fertility specialists during IVF procedures, where estrogen is used pre-transfer (to increase the lining of the uterus), will check the thyroid levels to make sure levels are not dropping. Often, giving thyroid medication at this time will ensure the levels stay steady.

Untreated thyroid conditions during pregnancy are linked to serious problems, including premature birth, miscarriage, and stillbirth.

Inadequately treated hypothyroidism has been associated with negative pregnancy outcomes. Thyroid hormone requirements increase with pregnancy, and many women with pre-existing hypothyroidism need an increase in their thyroid hormone doses in the first trimester of pregnancy.

The Endocrine Society recommends maintaining TSH levels from 0.2-<2.5 mU/L in the first trimester of pregnancy and between 0.3 to 3 mU/L in the remaining trimesters. This study examined the relationship between TSH levels in early pregnancy and the risk of adverse pregnancy outcomes.

Many women with hypothyroidism on thyroid hormone replacement therapy have TSH levels above the desired 2.5 mU/L level in early pregnancy. Higher TSH levels (TSH levels > 4.5 mU/L) are associated with an increased risk for miscarriage and should be avoided in early pregnancy.[32]

If Hashimoto's is present, thyroid peroxidase (TPO) levels will typically be elevated.

Values above 9.0 IU/mL generally are associated with autoimmune thyroiditis, but elevations are also seen in other autoimmune diseases.[33]

If you find out you have elevated levels of TPO and Hashimoto's that has been verified, it's important to change your diet and lifestyle as soon as possible to bring these levels down to protect your thyroid gland. Over time, by not making changes, the antibodies may attack your thyroid until it cannot do its job.

If you have elevated TPOs, address these areas:

- the correct medication to regulate hormones (a doctor will need to prescribe this)

- an anti-inflammatory diet (I recommend an anti-inflammatory Mediterranean diet to start with)

- regulation of the adrenal glands (testing is required to know what is needed)

- removing toxins both internally (diet) and from the home environment and balancing the gut flora and its lining (stool testing will reveal what treatment is needed for this)

Autoimmune hypothyroidism is a disease most commonly associated with POF (Premature Ovarian Failure), so screening by measurement of TSH, free T4, anti-thyroid-peroxidase and anti-thyroglobulin antibody levels is recommended. However, genetic factors, viral infection, other auto-immune disorders, as well as stress factors on the body and ovaries, may also play a part.

Premature ovarian failure (POF) is when a woman under 40 years old stops getting her period. It's caused by the ovaries not working properly, leading to low levels of important hormones (such as estrogen), so they can't typically have a baby. Treatment for this depends on the causative factor(s). Most often, couples with this diagnosis who wish to have a baby will be guided toward IVF, possibly using donor eggs, or adoption.

However, I would suggest getting a diagnosis first via testing. If tests show the issue is inflammation based, or due to other health factors other than genetics, there might be treatment options to help the ovaries work more efficiently.

Here are a few ways to reduce inflammation:

- Practice grounding. Grounding is where you walk or stand barefoot on the ground, whether it is dirt, grass, or sand. When you become "grounded" to the electron-enriched earth, you improve your sympathetic and parasympathetic nervous system balance.

- Being grounded cuts inflammation by thinning your blood and infusing your body with negatively charged ions, and many people have reported improvement in many ailments.

- Eliminate processed foods as well as foods that show sensitivities when tested.

- Avoid alcohol and processed sugar.

- Eat organic foods as much as possible and drink purified/filtered water.

- Take anti-inflammatory herbs and supplements.

See *Section 3* for more guidance on detoxing and supplemental advice.

ACTION PLAN

1. Get blood lab testing for liver markers (AST, ALT, GGT), blood glucose, HA1C, cortisol (at least for waking and before bedtime), and a lipid panel. A full panel with TSH, free T3, free T4, TPO, and TGA should be done to test the thyroid.

2. Dietary changes are important, such as eliminating sugars and processed foods. Do a big refrigerator and cabinet clean-up so you are not tempted.

3. Prep meals the night before for the next day's three meals and snacks. Pack balanced meals with a clean protein (nothing processed), a non-starchy vegetable or lettuce-based salad, and a small amount of starch—half a potato or yam, for instance. Good snack options would be fresh berries and nuts of choice.

4. Avoid bread and wheat products, as they are not easily digested and can negatively impact the thyroid (due to excess gluten and heavy pesticides).

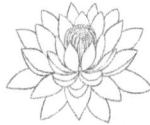

GENETIC *Impact* ON *Fertility*

"Our greatest glory is not in never falling,
but in rising every time we fall."

—CONFUCIUS

In the late 1990s, I went to a Resolve meeting (The National Infertility Association) where women having problems conceiving have a safe space to talk with each other and feel supported. I listened to one woman's story of how she had tried with her husband to conceive for a couple of years before trying in vitro fertilization (IVF).

Her story was sad because she went through seven IVF cycles before they investigated the couple's genetics. They found out that they both had the gene for cystic fibrosis in the same line, so that would mean that any child they conceived would likely have this challenging problem if the baby survived pregnancy and birth.

Spending that much money on IVF and the emotional roller coaster that goes with it, only to find out this outcome, is devastating. Not to mention the seven rounds of hormones and stimulants used with each IVF, as it can be rough on the body (especially after a few, let alone seven).

Fortunately, if you have already been to a fertility specialist, they will typically do genetic testing at the onset of care before any treatment. If more people knew that genetic risks could be a problem, they could avoid much of the frustration and heartache.

It is estimated that nearly 50% of infertility cases are due to genetic defects. I'm not saying everything has to do with genetics because it doesn't; however, knowing could be helpful, especially if you've been trying without success for a long time with the same partner.

WHY IS GENETIC TESTING IMPORTANT FOR FERTILITY?

Preconception carrier screening is a common genetic test for women and men planning a pregnancy. Carrier screening can determine whether you carry a genetic condition. Carriers of a genetic condition have one working and one nonworking copy of a particular gene.

Miscarriages due to genetic issues often occur before ten weeks of pregnancy. They are usually caused by random errors that cells make during normal cell division when the inherited instructions stored in the DNA don't function properly.[34]

This is often seen with advanced maternal aging and environmental chemicals that can damage genes and hormones. HPV (human papillomavirus) is an example of a mutagen that can affect reproduction, as well as Epstein-Barr virus, H-pylori, Hepatitis B and C, and anything that negatively impacts your DNA.

Some who carry chromosomal rearrangement may have never achieved a viable pregnancy if each previous conception resulted in a chromosomally unbalanced embryo that miscarried spontaneously.

Several genetic diseases can impact fertility in both men and women. If conception takes several years and you haven't been tested for genetics, this is a good time to do so.

If a genetic issue is not allowing your body to hold a pregnancy, there may be other solutions besides an IUI or IVF.

MTHFR (Methylenetetrahydrofolate Reductase)

The MTHFR gene mutation was discovered in 2003 because of the human genome project. These gene mutations, which can cause various health issues, have become more common.

The MTHFR gene instructs your body to make the MTHFR protein, which helps your body process folate. Your body needs folate to make DNA and modify proteins. When the MTHFR gene is affected in one parent (heterozygous) or both parents (homozygous), a higher amount of folate (not folic acid) is needed in the diet and with supplementation. The insufficiency can cause difficulties in becoming pregnant or maintaining a pregnancy if additional folate isn't added.[35]

Some other genetic patterns could be problematic for fertility but might have a reduced chance of passing them on to a baby in IVF. Knowing that a problem exists in the genetics, the embryologist may be able to carefully select the embryo that is unaffected by the following genetic diseases and then transfer the unaffected embryo.

Sickle Cell Anemia

Sickle cell anemia is a genetic disorder where the red blood cells become shaped like sickles or crescent moons instead of the usual round shape (referred to as sickling of blood cells). These abnormal cells can block blood flow, leading to pain, infections, and other complications. Sickle cell disease can affect fertility in males and females, but it is more common in males. The reproductive issues associated with sickle cell disease include:

For males:

- Delay in puberty (sexual maturation)
- Priapism (a painful erection that lasts for several hours)
- Primary gonad dysfunction
- Hypogonadism (a clinical syndrome associated with poor testosterone production, infertility, and erectile dysfunction)
- Abnormal spermatozoa indicating testicular dysfunction
- Abnormalities in the accessory sex organs, such as the seminal vesicles and the prostate gland, particularly given the marked decrease in ejaculate volume of the patients

For females:

- Lower ovarian reserve of follicles (which develop into eggs) than women without sickle cell disease, which can increase miscarriages, reduce fertility, and cause early menopause.

- Chronic inflammation, oxidative stress, and sickling of blood cells in the ovaries can make it harder for women to get pregnant.[36]

Hydroxyurea therapy, used to increase certain red blood cells called fetal hemoglobin, which may prevent the sickle-shaped red blood cells from forming, contributes to infertility in adult men with sickle cell disease.[37] However, it is unclear how sickle cell anemia directly affects fertility outcomes.

Couples with sickle cell trait may minimize the risk of having a child with sickle cell disease by pursuing in vitro fertilization with preimplantation genetic testing. For PGD, the couple must use in vitro fertilization. Preimplantation embryos are biopsied, and only the embryos without sickle cell anemia are selected.[38]

Cystic Fibrosis

Most women with cystic fibrosis (CF) are still fertile and can become pregnant. However, some may experience fertility problems due to thicker cervical mucus and ovulation issues caused by poor nutrition. Despite their thicker cervical mucus and possible ovulation issues, healthy women with CF often do not have compromised fertility and experience few physical barriers to becoming pregnant aside from having thicker cervical mucus.[39]

In contrast, men with CF usually produce normal levels of sex hormones such as progesterone, estrogen, and testosterone and can enjoy a normal sex life. However, the genetic mutation that causes CF results in infertility in almost all males. Ninety-eight percent of men with CF are infertile due to a blocked or missing vas deferens, which prevents the sperm from mixing with the semen.

In summary, while women with CF can experience fertility problems, most are still fertile and can become pregnant. Men with CF, on the other hand, are almost always infertile due to a blocked or missing vas deferens.

Thalassemia

Thalassemia, a genetic blood disorder where hemoglobin, the protein in the red blood cells that carries oxygen throughout the body is abnormally produced, can affect fertility in both men and women.

In women:

- Thalassemia can cause hormonal imbalances, leading to abnormal ovulation.

- Iron overload due to thalassemia can damage the pituitary gland, which regulates the activities of the ovaries, leading to infertility issues.

- Thalassemia can cause premature ovarian aging, which can lead to infertility sooner than in non-thalassemia patients.

In men:

- Thalassemia can cause hormonal imbalances that can lead to impaired sperm quality.

- Men with beta-thalassemia who receive regular blood transfusions are prone to developing acquired hypogonadism, which can lead to infertility.

- Thalassemia patients who undergo allogeneic hematopoietic stem cell transplantation (HSCT) have lower fertility potential, mainly in sperm parameters, compared with patients treated with blood transfusion and chelation.

Despite these challenges, both male and female thalassemic patients may conceive spontaneously, or conception may be achieved by assisted reproductive techniques (ART). Thalassemia patients must receive timely fertility care and take additional precautions like iron chelation injections to prevent iron overload.

With the development of advanced assisted reproductive techniques like IVF, the possibility of conceiving a healthy child despite thalassemia has increased.

Spinal Muscular Atrophy

Spinal muscular atrophy (SMA) is an inherited condition that causes muscle weakness and wasting due to the motor neurons in the spinal cord not working properly. SMA affects muscles throughout the body, including the muscles in the shoulders, hips, and back, which are often most severely affected, and the muscles for feeding and swallowing. SMA has no cure, but some promising treatments are being tested in clinical trials.

Research has shown that SMA adversely impacts male reproductive organ development and male fertility. However, there is no evidence to suggest that SMA affects female fertility.

Genetic testing can be very helpful in uncovering what may be the problem. However, genetic testing has some disadvantages and risks.[40]

- Increased stress and anxiety
- Results in some cases may return inconclusive or uncertain.
- Negative impact on family and personal relationships.
- You might not be eligible if you do not fit certain criteria required for testing.

ACTION PLAN

1. Have sperm and egg genetically tested by a fertility specialist.
2. Have a blood test for genetics for both of you to rule out any factors impacting your fertility.

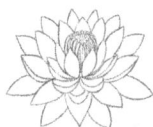

Gastrointestinal ISSUES AND *Immune* SENSITIVITIES: ARE THEY AFFECTING YOUR *Fertility?*

"A little progress each day
adds up to big results."

—ANONYMOUS

Sarah, at age 37, had been trying for one and a half years to conceive with her husband, John. She had become pregnant once, but unfortunately, it was an ectopic pregnancy (where the embryo attaches in the fallopian tube, which is dangerous, but when caught early, medication can release it without damaging the tube).

She came to me sad and frustrated, not knowing what to do differently to have the baby that she so desired. She was currently utilizing intrauterine insemination to see if it would increase their odds of conceiving, but so far, it hadn't happened.

Sarah struggled with irritable bowel syndrome, which caused diarrhea, heartburn, and burping often. She struggled to digest fatty foods because her gallbladder was removed; in fact, she noted that she was having more food issues lately that affected her digestion.

She was tired all the time and very stressed with her job. She'd had chlamydia in the past and struggled often with yeast infections. Her periods were light, lasting only two to three days of light to medium flow. She didn't notice any fertile cervical mucus at mid-cycle. She was experiencing night sweats and had low back pain and muscle twitching. Sleep was difficult, and her blood pressure ran low.

Her husband experienced stress as well as anxiety after serving several tours with the military. His sperm test revealed a low sperm count. He was given a multivitamin and other supplementation for his sperm and encouraged to have "talk therapy" with a specialist on the anxiety from his wartime experiences.

I focused her treatment on removing inflammatory factors, such as foods that might be causing more digestive difficulties. Running a food sensitivity test with the top 88 foods revealed quite a few sensitivities with foods she ate regularly. This constant irritation to her gastrointestinal tract can cause less absorption of nutrients and more inflammation near the reproductive organs.

Once we knew which foods she needed to avoid, we looked at other options for her meals that wouldn't upset the IBS. The plan included a good quality prenatal supplement, Chinese herbs to regulate and support her reproduction, and digestive enzymes, probiotics, and acupuncture to help digestion, lower inflammation, and support fertility.

She was hopeful that this treatment would be the answer to having a viable pregnancy that would bring them the child they both desired.

We continued treatment for close to eight months. She took a pregnancy test at that time … and it was positive! She and John were ecstatic, of course, especially since she didn't have to try an intrauterine insemination.

At seven weeks, her ultrasound revealed a strong heartbeat, with the embryo clearly in the uterus this time. Hearing the heartbeat and knowing that the baby would grow in the right place was wonderful and very reassuring.

Besides gastrointestinal issues such as IBS that Sarah struggled with, there are many others, including IBD, celiac disease, leaky gut, and SIBO.

Some common types of immune sensitivities that can lead to inflammation and should be addressed through testing (if unknown):

- Food sensitivities due to leaky gut
- Environmental sensitivities

- Chemical sensitivities
- Celiac disease
- Endometriosis
- Small intestine bacterial overgrowth (SIBO)

Let's look at some of the more common health issues that can create problems with nutrient absorption due to leaky gut causing food sensitivities, which can lead to inflammation. It's much more common than most people realize.

Intolerances and sensitivities are different but are still immune responses. Your body sees these invaders, such as food chemicals, as it would a virus or bacteria inside a cell; they attach to the cell and either engulf or destroy it.

Food sensitivities create chronic low-level inflammation. They can cause leaky gut and have been associated with damage to the fallopian tubes and ovaries.

One thing to consider is the proximity of the intestinal organs and urinary bladder to the uterus, fallopian tubes, and ovaries. They are all "smushed" together, so it's easy to see how inflammation in the gastrointestinal system and bladder can affect your reproductive organs.

Here are just a few of the chemicals released by your immune system when you are suffering from food or chemical sensitivities or intolerances and the different symptoms that could be experienced:

Prostaglandins: Pain, shortness of breath, fast heart rate/heart palpitations, flushing, diarrhea, abdominal cramps.

Histamines: Headaches, itching, burning sensations, crampy abdominal pain, a general sense of anxiety with deep, "odd" body sensations. Patients sometimes say, "I feel weird all over" or complain of a "... deep, pricking, or crawling sensation ..."

Cytokines: Fever, sense of impending doom, memory loss, brain fog, headaches, loss of appetite, difficulty swallowing, sleepiness, fatigue, depression, and anxiety.

Disruptions in female reproductive functions by endocrine-disrupting chemicals may result in sub-fertility, infertility, improper hormone production, estrous and menstrual cycle abnormalities, anovulation (not ovulating), and early reproductive senescence.[41]

With celiac disease, although it produces a different autoimmune reaction against wheat and gluten-containing grains, rye, oats, and barley than IgG-mediated food sensitivities, it can have the same effect on reducing fertility in both men and women.

As mentioned before, in food sensitivities, the toxins can increase the hormone prolactin, which has been associated with celiac disease and other gluten reactions.

Celiac in males has been shown to affect sperm shape. Sperm carry half of the DNA for a female egg to be fertilized, so healthy sperm plays a crucial role in conception as well as the risk for miscarriages.

Over the last 10 years, several studies have found conflicting results when looking at the link between celiac disease and infertility. Some studies have found that women with undiagnosed celiac disease may have issues with fertility, while others have shown that there is no increased risk of infertility.

Celiac disease can be tested by a GI doctor, integrative doctor, or Certified Functional Medicine practitioner. If you are not sure if your gastrointestinal symptoms are gluten or wheat-based, then having a test done for food sensitivity for gliadins (wheat gluten, as well as rye, spelt, and barley) will let you know if you should be avoiding gluten/gliadin-based grains.

It is not known if the nutritional issues (malabsorption) that occur with untreated celiac disease may cause reproductive issues or if the immune system may be to blame.

However, a recent study published in *Human Reproduction* shows how critical it is for physicians to consider undiagnosed celiac disease when a woman has reproductive problems.

The study found that when women with celiac disease were undiagnosed, they had 11 more miscarriages per 1,000 pregnancies and 1.62 more stillbirths per 1,000 pregnancies.

In the two years before celiac disease diagnosis, women also become pregnant less often, with 25 fewer pregnancies per 1,000. The overall risk of pregnancy problems in undiagnosed women was 15 more per 1,000 pregnancies compared to women who did not have celiac disease.

The conclusion was that undiagnosed celiac disease can lead to stillbirths and miscarriages, but diagnosis makes a difference.

Other results found are as follows:

Celiac Disease, Infertility, and Women

- Some researchers have found that the prevalence of celiac disease in women with unexplained fertility is higher than in the general population.
- Evidence suggests that women with undiagnosed celiac disease have an increased risk of pre-term birth and spontaneous miscarriage.
- Studies have shown that women with celiac disease have an increased risk for polycystic ovarian syndrome and endometriosis.
- Many celiac disease experts recommend that women with unexplained infertility be screened for celiac disease.[42]

Non-Celiac Gluten Sensitivity (NCGS) and Infertility

There is a lack of scientific information and research studies on the potential link between non-celiac gluten sensitivity (NCGS, also commonly referred to as "gluten intolerance") and infertility. While research needs to be done, those with non-celiac gluten sensitivity are thought to possibly be at an increased risk of reproductive issues. One case review did suggest that a strict gluten-free diet may improve fertility for those with NCGS.[43]

Being "gluten-free" means avoiding all gliadin-based options, not just wheat-based products. The list would include spelt, rye, barley, wheat, and oats (with oats, they might be okay if not run through a mill with other gluten-based foods in it). They can't claim to be gluten-free if this is the case.

Small Intestine Bacterial Overgrowth (SIBO)

Small intestinal bacterial overgrowth (SIBO) is defined as the presence of excessive bacteria in the small intestine. Recent findings link the cause to food poisoning at some point, maybe not even a severe case, just enough to put bacteria in an area where it shouldn't be.

The presence of increasing numbers of the bacteria Klebsiella and E. coli can upset the balance needed in the small intestine to help absorb nutrients from foods. This overgrowth is frequently implicated as the cause of chronic diarrhea and malabsorption.

However, it could be due to having low stomach acid, poor gut motility (ability to move digested food through to the large intestine), or using certain medications (any that might lower stomach acids or slow bowel transit might cause or add to the condition).

It has been found that those with autoimmune diseases like Crohn's and celiac disease are at a higher risk for SIBO.

Three different gases tend to increase due to higher bacteria levels: hydrogen, hydrogen sulfide, and methane.[44]

Hydrogen-dominant SIBO is characterized by bacteria in the small intestine that produces hydrogen gas. This is the most common type.

Hydrogen sulfide SIBO occurs when bacteria in the small intestine consume the hydrogen gas made by other bacteria to produce hydrogen sulfide, which smells like rotten eggs. This type of SIBO may cause diarrhea.

Methane-dominant SIBO is characterized by an overgrowth of methane-producing bacteria in the small intestine. This SIBO type is associated with constipation.

Mixed SIBO occurs when hydrogen and methane gas are elevated with a SIBO breath test, suggesting overgrowth of both methane-producing and hydrogen-producing bacteria.

Some of the common symptoms are abdominal pain; bloating; gas; constipation, diarrhea, or both; heartburn; nausea; carbohydrate intolerance; malabsorption; nutrient deficiencies; stress and anxiety; brain fog; and joint pain.

Testing requires a two- or three-hour home breath test. However, the most reliable tests must be ordered by an Integrative Medicine MD, Functional Medicine Practitioner, or Naturopath, who utilizes testing for all three types of gases, as not all labs will do this.

If you do test positive for SIBO, it's important to go through a program specifically designed to get rid of the overgrowth of bacteria in the small intestine before trying to conceive.

If you test positive for SIBO before trying to conceive, the following steps can be taken:

1. Consult a doctor: If you have signs and symptoms that are common to SIBO, make an appointment with your doctor. After an initial evaluation, you may be referred to a doctor specializing in treatment.

2. Diagnosis: To diagnose SIBO, you may have tests to check for bacterial overgrowth in your small intestine, poor fat absorption, or other problems that may be causing your symptoms. Tests for SIBO include small intestine aspirate and fluid culture, breath tests, blood tests, and stool tests.

3. Treatment: For most people, the initial way to treat bacterial overgrowth is with antibiotics. Doctors may start this treatment if your symptoms and medical history strongly suggest this is the cause, even when test results are inconclusive or without any testing. Testing may be performed if antibiotic treatment is not effective. If you can't identify or fix the underlying cause, you can try to manage bacterial overgrowth with a low-carb diet and probiotics.

ACTION PLAN

1. It is important to consult a doctor and follow their advice before trying to conceive if you test positive for SIBO.

2. Look for a GI specialist who checks for all three types of SIBO and does at least a two-hour test, but a three-hour would be better.

3. If you test positive, you will need to go through a clearing either with antibiotics or with a holistic practitioner using herbal antibiotic blends and other ways to balance out the gut microbiome.

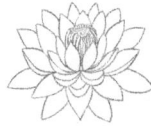

MALE FACTOR
Infertility

"Just keep swimming."

—DORY, FINDING NEMO

I'm often amazed by how few tests were performed with the male patients that I've seen or who have been told their sperm analysis was good enough, so no other tests were necessary. Or the other scenario where only the woman came for fertility treatment, but the husband wasn't tested at all (no sperm analysis, no hormone tests, or overall health assessment).

Male factors account for at least 50% of all infertility cases worldwide. Some factors such as radiation, smoking, a varicocele, infection, urinary tract infection, environmental factors, nutritional deficiencies, and oxidative stress contribute to male infertility.

I strongly urge women that I see to urge their partners to be thoroughly tested to rule out sperm abnormalities, genetic issues, hormonal irregularities, or other health-related issues that could impact their fertility.

Men need to do their part too. It's unfortunate when the woman is seen for many months or years and has been tested, and they don't know why she hasn't conceived, only to have the partner finally agree to test and find the issue is with his sperm.

This is not to say this is always the case, as it isn't, but ruling it out saves time and often the considerable stress the woman holds onto, thinking it is all on her to conceive.

Some of the male infertility-related factors are as follows:

- Unknown or "unexplained" infertility
- 40-50% of infertility is related to male factors
- Low sperm count and volume
- Poor morphology
- Low motility
- Anti-sperm antibodies
- DNA fragmentation in sperm doubles from ages 30-45

A low sperm count refers to an abnormally reduced number of sperm in the ejaculate, and it can cause problems in conception. Western medicine believes this condition to be due to decreased sperm production from a varicocele or one of the following:

- Medications (alpha-blockers for blood pressure)
- Low testosterone levels (or too high if taking testosterone medication)
- Alcohol, tobacco, and drug usage
- A very high level of stress or depression
- Chromosomal issues, tumors, or surgeries (reverse vasectomies, spinal, prostate or bladder surgeries)
- Weight gain (affects hormones that can reduce fertility)
- Hormone imbalances (hypothalamus, pituitary, testicles, thyroid, or adrenals)
- Undescended testicles or mumps, or an STD
- Problems with ejaculation (retrograde or lack of ejaculation, erectile dysfunction)
- Celiac disease (need to have a gluten-free diet)

WHAT TESTING IS NECESSARY

Men need a thorough evaluation of their hormones as well as a comprehensive sperm analysis w/Kruger strict criterion.

In the fifth edition of the WHO manual, the Kruger strict criteria require normal sperm to be measured for head size and determine that if any one structural feature (head, appearance, width, length, neck, or tail) has a defect, then the sperm are considered to be abnormally formed.[45]

An abnormally shaped sperm can fertilize an egg, and having abnormally shaped sperm does not necessarily mean you will be completely unable to fertilize an egg, but even when a man has a normal sperm count and sperm motility, some defects in sperm morphology may make it take longer to achieve pregnancy or even prevent it.

Usually, men will need their primary physician to refer them to a urologist for a sperm analysis and a physical to make sure there aren't any issues with their reproductive organs (a varicocele being present or another issue).

- For hormone testing, they will typically be referred to a reproductive endocrinologist.

- Having a comprehensive blood lab test could help verify if any other health issues could be problematic to their fertility. (Ruling out issues such as diabetes, hypothyroid, inflammation, fatty liver, etc.)

- Hormone testing should include both total and free testosterone, total estrogens, progesterone, DHEA, sex hormone binding globulin (SHBG), follicle-stimulating hormone (FSH), luteinizing hormone (LH), and a thyroid panel (TSH, free T3, free T4, and thyroid antibodies).

Hormone tests would be recommended if there are abnormal findings with the sperm analysis or there is low libido and energy, problems maintaining an erection, etc.

- Blood test for HA1C, fasting insulin, CRP, homocysteine levels, RBC with differential, and STDs.

- Genetic testing can also be beneficial as men can also have MTH-FR-related issues and more that can affect fertility.

The following shows what a sperm analysis should test for and their normal levels.

- Sperm volume (more than 1ml)

- Sperm density & total sperm count (more than 20 million per ml)

- Morphology (<30% normally shaped)

- Motility (<50% actively motile)
- Liquification time: 20-30 min after collection
- Anti-sperm antibodies (negative findings)
- PH: 7.12-8.00

A Sperm Chromatin Structure Assay (through SCSA Diagnostics for around $500 but may be covered by insurance) can check for chromosomal damage to the DNA of sperm.

WHAT IS A VARICOCELE, AND HOW WOULD I KNOW IF I HAVE ONE?

A varicocele is when local veins in either one testicle or both are enlarged, twisted, and protruded, which can cause blood pooling in the area and heat, which may harm sperm.

In mild cases, it can be asymptomatic. More typically, walking or standing for long periods can irritate the varicocele, while lying down may help to relieve the pain. If the condition is more severe, there may be a heavy sensation and pain in the scrotum and lower abdomen.

The increased temperatures can result in fewer sperm cells maturing, and those that do mature may have less motility or be malformed. (On a side note, this is one of the main reasons hot tubs aren't recommended when you are TTC.)

When you go to your urologist for a sperm analysis, they can determine if there is a varicocele.

WHEN THERE ARE NO SPERM PRESENT IN THE ANALYSIS

If you have a sperm analysis done and it shows that you don't have any sperm, the most obvious cause would be from a vasectomy. Still, it is more likely due to unstudied factors, such as genetic conditions, poor testicular development as a fetus or child, or environmental toxins.

I have seen this with failed reverse vasectomies, but I had another patient who was taking testosterone shots to help his low energy and libido, and it caused his body to completely stop producing sperm as a result. If I hadn't had him do a sperm analysis, he would have assumed that all was well. After he stopped the testosterone shots and instead took a fertility-enhancing herbal blend to raise his energy level and libido, his sperm count came back to normal, and they were able to conceive and have their baby!

There are therapies, supplements, and herbs that help correct many sperm abnormalities or deficiencies. No sperm present can be caused by different things, as mentioned, whether it's due to structural abnormalities, a blockage, or the use of testosterone, to name a few. It's always better to find out what's causing it and see if there's a fix.

The shape of sperm can affect fertility. When there are structural abnormalities, such as thickened sperm, it may be due to a varicocele or localized inflammation. If the sperm is too thick, it can affect its movement in the female reproductive tract. This can be seen in conditions like a reverse vasectomy. In simpler terms, the shape of the sperm can sometimes be different, and when this happens, it might make it harder for the sperm to move and fertilize an egg.[46]

THE ENDOCRINE SYSTEM

Endocrine glands, distributed throughout the body, produce the hormones that act as signaling molecules after release into the circulatory system. The human body depends on hormones for a healthy endocrine system, which controls many biological processes like normal growth, fertility, and reproduction. Hormones act in extremely small amounts, and minor disruptions in those levels may cause significant developmental and biological effects.

Some of these disruptors are present in numerous common items like cosmetics, food packaging, toys, carpets, and pesticides. Certain flame retardant chemicals can also act as endocrine disruptors. Exposure to these chemicals can happen through the air, food, skin, and water. Avoiding or eliminating EDCs completely is challenging, but you can make informed decisions to lower exposure and minimize potential health risks.[47]

In men, follicle-stimulating hormone acts on the Sertoli cells of the testes to stimulate sperm production, so it makes sense to test this if the sperm analysis shows a low sperm count (fewer than 15 million). FSH is the best indicator of the testes' sperm-making ability. FSH also maintains sperm until they are ready to be released, making it an essential hormone for fertility.

A normal level of FSH should be 1.5–12.4IU/L. (It is better below 7.0IU/L as higher levels can mean that the testes aren't functioning properly, so the pituitary goes into overdrive trying to stimulate them.)

Luteinizing hormone stimulates the production of testosterone from Leydig cells in the testes. Normal levels should be 1.24–7.8 IU/L (If too low, it can indicate a pituitary gland issue.)

Estradiol, the most common form of estrogen, is especially crucial to male sexuality. Testosterone is the most significant hormone in male sexual development and function, but estrogen needs to stay in balance with testosterone to help control sex drive, the ability to have an erection, and the production of sperm.[48]

Testosterone naturally decreases as men age, while estrogen increases. You don't need to be concerned about this unless your estrogen levels are abnormally high; this can be a risk factor for conditions like diabetes and certain forms of cancer.[49]

There are two main types of estrogen in men: estrone and estradiol. An adult male's average levels for estrone are 10–60 pg/ml and estradiol 10–40 pg/ml.

The main fertility symptoms of concern with having high estrogen levels in men are:

- **Infertility**. Estrogen is one of the hormones your body uses to produce sperm. High estrogen levels can slow down sperm production and make it harder to create healthy sperm.

- **Erectile dysfunction (ED)**. Increased estrogen levels can affect the balance of hormones that are needed to help get an erection and stay erect. This is especially true if you also experience low testosterone.[50]

Signs of high estrogen in men: reduced sex drive, reduced sperm concentration in semen, feeling exhausted, losing hair all over your body, shrinking muscle mass, reduced growth of penis and testicles, loss of bone density (osteoporosis), hot flashes, and having trouble focusing.

A diet that is low in fat and high in fiber is recommended when estrogen levels are high. Follow these recommendations until estrogen levels normalize:

- Eat cruciferous vegetables (including broccoli, cauliflower, cabbage, and Brussels sprouts) containing phytochemicals that block estrogen production.

- Include shiitake and portobello mushrooms, which block estrogens in the body.

- Green tea is another good source of polyphenols.

- Pomegranates are high in estrogen-blocking phytochemicals.

- Eat only grass-fed meats and avoid those with added hormones.

- Avoid using plastic containers for food storage as they are hormone disruptors.

- Avoid any products that have parabens (they contain estrogens), such as shampoos.

- D.I.M. and Calcium D-Glucarate can also decrease high estrogen levels.

- Get regular exercise.

- DHEA supplementation may be needed if testing is showing a low level.

DHEA and DHEA-S are important for the body's production of the male sex hormone testosterone, which is crucial for normal sperm development. When there's a disorder leading to low testosterone, it can result in infertility.

It's important to test serum levels of both testosterone and DHEA to note whether they're low.

ELEVATED LEVELS OF HA1C (HEMOGLOBIN A1C)

A recent study of men attending a fertility clinic found that men suspected of prediabetes (abnormally high blood sugars) had higher levels of damage to sperm DNA, were more likely to have unexplained azoospermia (no sperm in the ejaculate) and had lower testosterone levels and more disruption of other fertility hormones, compared to men attending the clinic without clinical signs of prediabetes.[51]

Diabetes can damage blood vessels and nerves and increase the risk of infection, especially when not well controlled. It is associated with a range of sexual problems, including erectile dysfunction, decreased sex drive (libido), ejaculation problems, and inflammation of the foreskin (balanitis).

HA1C is a marker for insulin resistance, which can be considered prediabetes. HA1C levels are considered optimal if they are between 4.8 and 5.6. Levels between 5.7 and 6.4 would mean that you're prediabetic.

Supplements that can positively affect male fertility:

- Omega-3: 3gm a day to help sperm integrity and lessen inflammation.

- CO-Q-10: 200mg, 2 times a day for better morphology and sperm count (unless anxious)

- Alpha lipoic acid: 600mg per day could improve motility, reduce sperm DNA damage, and regulate high blood sugar.

- N-acetyl cysteine: 600mg per day lowers morphology and boosts testosterone.

- Methylfolate (1.2mg) w/ B12 (3mg): the dosage of folate would be higher if MTHFR is a factor (with either A1289C or C677T).

- L-Carnitine: 2gm a day for better motility and morphology.

- Vitamin C: 2000mg a day to reduce sperm DNA damage.

- Vitamin E: 400 IU a day for better morphology.

- To increase sperm count, eat more sesame seeds, almonds, flax seeds, pumpkin seeds, olives, avocados, and quinoa.

- Ginseng (Siberian): to increase testosterone.

- Zinc picolinate: 30mg.

- Selenomethionine: 200mcg per day.

- Decaf green or rooibos tea: for men with a high degree of DNA fragmentation.

In addition, there are male fertility formulas that contain many of the above supplements, so not so many different pills need to be taken.

Low levels of folate have been associated with a decreased sperm count and decreased sperm motility. In a recent study, combining zinc and folic acid (folate) resulted in a 75% increase in total normal sperm count in subfertile men.[52]

SIX FOODS TO AVOID FOR BEST FERTILITY

1. Fried foods—They may decrease sperm quality.

2. Full-fat dairy—Full-fat dairy contains estrogen and can lower healthy sperm. Opt for almond milk or other nut milk, or milk from grass-fed cows.

3. Processed meats—Processed meats (including bacon, ham, sausage, hot dogs, corned beef, beef jerky, canned meat, and meat sauces) can lower sperm count.

4. Caffeine—Researchers have linked caffeine consumption by both men and women in the weeks leading up to conception to an increased risk for miscarriage.

5. Alcohol—One or two alcoholic drinks are okay per week, but more than 14 mixed drinks in a week can lower testosterone levels and affect sperm count.

6. Cannabis (w/THC)—heavy use lowers sperm counts, decreases sperm motility (basically, their ability to swim), and increases sperm malformation (morphology). In very small quantities, it can be okay.[53]

ACTION PLAN

1. Make an appointment to see a urologist if you haven't done that yet. You may need a referral from your GP.

2. The urologist will be able to check for any structural issues, such as varicocele or other issues, and will do the sperm analysis as well.

3. Get on a good multivitamin and other supplementation that fits the findings.

4. Since it takes about 70 days for new sperm to be regenerated, you'll want to wait to retest after you make dietary, supplemental, and lifestyle changes for at least that period. Fever and heat to the testes can cause damage, so if they occur before retesting, wait another 70 days before TTC again.

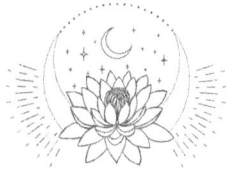

IMPORTANT
Changes
TO IMPROVE FERTILITY

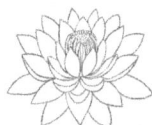

$\mathcal{D}\text{etoxing}$ YOUR HOME AND BODY

"As long as we are persistent in our pursuit of
our deepest destiny, we will continue to grow.

We cannot choose the day or time
when we will fully bloom.

It happens on its own."

—DENIS WAITLEY

Miranda came to see me because she was feeling really sick and couldn't figure out the cause. She was very frustrated, not knowing why she was feeling this way. She'd always been active, into sports and taking trips. This setback with her health was getting in the way of all of that and causing issues at home.

She had been living in an apartment with her husband when black mold was found, via testing, to be growing in her bathroom. She was having respiratory symptoms at the time, sinus congestion, and allergies, as well as worsening digestive problems (she'd had some digestive problems most of her life). To make matters worse, she unknowingly ingested mold when she ate a piece of fruit that didn't taste right. She was tested for blood mycotoxins, and several showed high levels.

Her other symptoms were regular yeast infections, elevated testosterone-causing acne, and a history of UTIs, which she had treated with rounds of antibiotics. She was very fatigued, and her vision was more blurred when tired. She noted hair loss, brittle nails, insomnia, and a lack of concentration, and her skin was peeling.

Besides testing for mycotoxins, she had a stool culture and a comprehensive blood panel done. She had had other tests done prior that revealed genetic issues of methylating, which can make healing more difficult unless she has the proper supplementation. Testing also showed that her thyroid was affected, especially with converting into T3, which helps your metabolism work effectively.

She had been on the NuvaRing but knew in a couple of years that she'd want to try to conceive. With all the health problems she was having, they would need to be corrected for her reproductive system to work well to be able to conceive and hold a pregnancy.

Unfortunately, further testing showed that she had Lyme disease. She went through a lot of internal "cleanup" to get the Lyme disease reduced so that she felt better, as her system was already in a deficit. With all of this on her plate, she was fortunately very tenacious and did all that was recommended by her Lyme doctor and me.

She did end up conceiving and having a baby in the next three years, but her system is still working hard postpartum to get back to normal.

WATCH OUT FOR TOXINS

Human fertility is declining worldwide. While much of the 50% decrease in the number of children born per woman in the past 60 years is due to choice, an increasing number of couples—now 1 in 7 to 10 in North America—are having a hard time getting pregnant, due in part to the increasing amount of harmful substances in the environment.[54]

Environmental toxins can cause infertility by disrupting the endocrine system, damaging the male or female reproduction cycle, or impairing the viability of the fetus. Many studies are finding a link between the recent increase in male infertility and the increased occurrence of mycotoxins (mold in food, homes, and buildings, as well as the environment.)[55]

This damage decreases natural fertility and makes in vitro fertilization (IVF) much less likely to succeed. The most harmful fertility disruptors are organochlorine compounds (chlorinated pesticides, polychlorinated biphenyls, and dioxins), bisphenol A (BPA), and organophosphate pesticides and herbicides. In addition, many other chemicals, metals, and air pollutants can seriously inhibit fertility.[56]

These are the main offenders to watch for in your diet and home:

Polychlorinated biphenyls (PCBs): Fluorescent light ballasts, thermal insulation material (including fiberglass, felt, foam, and cork), adhesives and tapes, oil-based paint, caulking, plastics, carbonless copy paper, floor finish, and more. They are suspected to affect male and female reproductive functions adversely.

Phthalates: These are a group of chemicals used in hundreds of products, such as toys, vinyl flooring and wall covering, detergents, lubricating oils, food packaging, pharmaceuticals, blood bags and tubing, and personal care products, such as nail polish, hair sprays, aftershave lotions, soaps, shampoos, perfumes, and other artificially scented products. Phthalates may induce alterations in puberty, the development of testicular dysgenesis syndrome, cancer, and fertility disorders in both males and females. At the hormonal level, phthalates can modify the release of hypothalamic, pituitary, and peripheral hormones.

Bisphenol A (BPA): This is found in polycarbonate plastics and epoxy resins. Polycarbonate plastics, such as water bottles, are often used in food and beverage containers. They are also found on grocery store receipts. Even the plastics that say they're BPA-free are variations and still cause harm. It's better to avoid plastics as much as possible.

There is increasing evidence that BPA has an impact on human fertility and is responsible for reproductive problems such as testicular dysgenesis syndrome, cryptorchidism, cancers, decreased fertility in males, and follicle loss in females.

Mercury: Fish with high mercury levels include king mackerel, shark, swordfish, marlin, orange roughy, and bigeye tuna. Limit these fish when you are attempting to conceive.

Thallium: This environmental toxic can cross the placental barrier during pregnancy, inducing inflammation. It is found in water and foods (higher concentrations have been found in kale, even in organic kale, so watch your intake).

Lead and cadmium: These heavy metals are known to be potential female reproductive toxins.[57] Experimental data have revealed that exposure to cadmium affects female fertility by altering ovulation, steroid synthesis, pituitary function, and fertilization.

Electromagnetic fields (cells & laptops): From currently available studies, it is clear that radiofrequency electromagnetic fields (RF-EMF) have adverse effects on sperm, such as sperm count, size and shape, and motility.

These lists can seem overwhelming, as it's challenging to completely avoid all of the toxins listed here. But this is about minimizing your exposure to the toxins in your home environment where you have the most control.

Detoxification, or cleaning the house inside and out, can help your hormones and body systems, including your reproductive system, function more efficiently. Reduction, if not complete elimination, is key. Dietary changes are crucial to help your body clear out many toxic contaminants: switching to organic foods and products, keeping sugars out of the diet, only one cup of mycotoxin-free coffee daily, grass-fed meats, cold water caught fish, and avoiding alcohol, marijuana, and other drugs.

Detoxification is an important first step. No matter how long you've been trying to conceive, clearing the liver of toxins that have accumulated, which negatively impact hormonal conversion, will help you over the next 90 days. It takes that long for your body to make the egg that will be ovulated (called the Graafian follicle).

There are so many environmental toxins around us consistently. As time passes, more and more toxins and chemicals are being used in our food, drinks, water, skincare, work and home environments, and basically, everywhere we go.

You are subjected to "toxins" in your:

- Fruits, vegetables, meats, and processed foods (via pesticides, fungicides, insecticides)
- Bath & beauty products (anything with artificial fragrance, parabens, and more)
- Cleaning supplies (both for home and commercial use)
- The plastics that we use to contain our food in the refrigerator and freezer and on paper receipts from stores.
- Pollution from big industry that we breathe in each day, and more!

It's impossible to avoid every toxin around you daily, but you can do things in your home to limit your daily intake.

There are several ways to test for toxic overload and heavy metal exposure. Whether you have a hair analysis, urinalysis, or blood draw, they can all reveal toxicity levels, whether by chemicals or heavy metal burden.

Here are other things you can do:

1. Eat organically grown foods as much as possible (refer to the Dirty Dozen and Clean 15 recommendations in the next chapter) and avoid processed foods.

2. Make your cleaning products (or buy from the "safe" list in the bonus section).

3. Use organic skincare products that don't contain anything on the toxin list.

CLEANING UP YOUR HOME ENVIRONMENT

Detoxifying your home is a holistic approach to eliminating harmful elements that affect every area of your life, from the air you breathe to the products you use or don't use. You might be surprised at some of the places where toxins hide.

- Get rid of all plastic containers and switch to Pyrex or another type of glass container that is freezer-safe. (Freezing or microwaving plastic releases BPA and other toxins into your food that are endocrine disruptors.)

- Get a good water filter for your drinking water that will leach out lead, chlorine, other heavy minerals, and toxins, as well as fluoride (if possible). Use a shower filter as well for bathing, as that water is absorbed into your skin.

- Paper receipts have BPA on them, so ask for emailed receipts whenever possible.

- Avoid Roundup/Glyphosate spraying and using it around your home.

- Avoid bug sprays; instead, try a vinegar/water spray around areas or essential oil sprays with water, such as a peppermint/water mix, lavender/eucalyptus, or citronella.

- If you are around strong paints, lacquers, etc., wear a mask and gloves.

A detox is a very good idea before trying to conceive, and it's never too late to thoroughly clean up what's in your kitchen cupboards and refrigerator. Then, with your partner, do at least a two-week cleanse to lower toxins and inflammation from processed foods, drinks, and the environment.

I offer a free two-week detox plan on my site that is good for both men and women. (See Resources for more help.)

ACTION PLAN (TWO-WEEK CLEANSE)

1. Stop drinking alcohol, coffee, sodas, and caffeinated drinks, and avoid all processed foods.

2. Don't smoke or use any drugs (this includes pain relievers, if possible) unless it is a prescribed drug that is not on the avoidance list.

3. Only eat organic fruits and vegetables, grass-fed meat, cold water-caught fish, and non-hormone antibiotic-free chicken. Vegetable and chicken broths are good, as well as beans, nuts, and seeds. Avoid any foods that are irritating or to which you have a known allergy.

4. You can have herbal teas such as peppermint, dandelion, nettles, decaf chai tea, and decaf green tea.

5. If it's herbal tea, it will count toward your daily water intake. Look into getting a good reverse osmosis system for your home or at least one that you can connect to the kitchen faucet. In the resource section, I've included a two-week cleanse that you can use for guidance.

6. Drink purified water only. If you're not at home, use a stainless-steel drinking bottle; do not use plastic. The amount of purified water you'll want to drink daily is determined based on your weight. Plan to drink half of your body weight in ounces. (For example, if you weigh 140 lbs, you'll need to drink 70 oz. of water daily.)

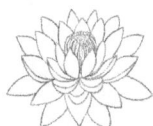

DIET AND SUPPLEMENTATION FOR
Fertility

"Whatever the struggle, continue the climb.
It may be only one step to the summit."

—DIANE WESTLAKE

There are so many things that can be done to encourage the good health of your body and reproductive system, and many areas where you may be having a negative effect on creating an optimum healthy environment.

For instance, there are certain medications that can impact fertility. To check on the ones that you are currently taking, you can go to drug.com and search for your medications. I think the easier way to find specifics relating to fertility is to do a Google search and ask, "Does [fill in your medication here] negatively affect fertility in males or females?"

If you're prescribed a medication that is considered necessary, ask your doctor for a different medication, if possible, that won't impact your fertility.

Another area that is key for optimum fertility is your nutrition. Doing a thorough review of your daily diet choices, drinking, sweets, and other vices is a good idea.

I'm a big fan of the 80-20 rule. It means that 80% of the time, you are eating healthy and taking good care of yourself. The other 20% of the time, you allow yourself a little treat. It's a good way to take care of your health while still allowing for your favorite food, etc., without feeling like you're "missing out."

The problem is that many of us live our lives with the inverse option of 80% treats and unhealthy choices and only 20% healthy options. When stress is constant in our lives, it's easy to go for "comfort foods," which all too often fall under "unhealthy options."

Diet is extremely important for optimizing your fertility! If you're eating from the wrong isles of the market, changing that now will help.

Find a health food store in your area that offers a good array of organic produce to choose from, as well as healthier options for snack foods. However, even with a health food store, you'll be better off sticking to the "outer aisles" where you can find organic fruits and vegetables, grass-fed meats, organic cage-free chicken, and cold-water-caught fish.

The inner aisles mean bringing your "readers" so you can pay attention to the very small print regarding the ingredients and fillers. Even at health food stores, there are still preservatives and bad ingredients in some products.

Also, I strongly advise you to make a list of foods that you need for the week. The list should include beautiful leafy greens for salads and to add to smoothies or soup if time is an issue (be sure the list of ingredients on cans is short and you recognize what they are; a long list may mean some hidden or not-so-healthy options). But if you're shopping at places like Trader Joe's, Jimbo's, Whole Foods, and even some Costco's, then you will normally have a lot of healthy options to choose from.

I'm a big fan of the anti-inflammatory Mediterranean diet. It includes lots of fruits and vegetables, nuts, legumes, some grains, and fish, with lesser amounts of meat. I prefer to leave out gluten products as much as possible, mainly because they have been heavily sprayed with pesticides, which increase inflammation in the body, as we weren't made to deal with this and other types of toxins, especially when so much is added to our foods, drinks, and more.

Grocery Store Checklist:

- Fresh vegetables like tomatoes, cabbage, okra, edamame, and carrots
- Leafy greens like romaine lettuce, spinach, bok choy, endive, arugula, and radicchio
- Canned vegetables, if necessary; make sure that they are low in sodium
- Frozen vegetables like broccoli or cauliflower without added butter or sauces
- Fresh fruits like apples, oranges, bananas, mangoes, guava, and papaya
- Canned, frozen, or dried fruit without added sugars
- Berries like raspberries, blueberries, blackberries, and strawberries
- Seafood like fish and shellfish
- Hormone and cage-free poultry like chicken or turkey breast without skin or lean ground chicken or turkey (at least 93% lean)
- Grass-fed meats: meats that come from animals that have been fed a diet of grass and other forage, rather than grains like corn and soy that are harder to digest
- Beans, peas, and lentils like black beans and garbanzo beans (chickpeas)
- Eggs from chickens that are cage-free
- Unsalted nuts, seeds, and nut butter like almond or peanut butter
- Tempeh-vegan protein option
- Healthy fats and oils like organic olive and/or avocado

Farmer's markets are great places to buy vegetables and fruits that are in season, and they often have organic and grass-fed options. When shopping for grains, look for quinoa, oats, buckwheat (which contains no wheat), and other wheat-free options like lentils.

Additionally, consider adding coconut milk to your list, which is a great dairy-free alternative. Finally, don't forget to drink plenty of water and unsweetened coconut water. Avoid sugary drinks as much as possible; instead, try slightly diluted fruit juices.

For those doubting pesticides' effect on your produce and why buying organic is a good idea, please read the results of the following studies.

Several studies have investigated the effects of fertility from pesticide residue on fruits and vegetables, and the results suggest that there may be a negative association between the two. Here are some key findings from the search results:

- A study published in *JAMA Internal Medicine* found that women who ate more than two servings of high-pesticide fruits or vegetables each day were 18% less likely to become pregnant and 26% less likely to have a live birth than women with the lowest exposure.[58]

- Another study published in the same journal found that intake of high-pesticide residue fruits and vegetables was associated with lower probabilities of clinical pregnancy and live birth among women undergoing infertility treatment with assisted reproductive technology.

- A study from Harvard T.H. Chan School of Public Health also found that eating fruits and vegetables with high amounts of pesticide residue, such as strawberries, spinach, peppers, or grapes, may reduce women's chances of conceiving and bearing children.[59]

- Pesticides on fruits and vegetables may lower the chances of a live birth in women who are being treated with IVF.

Based on these findings, it may be advisable for women trying to conceive to limit their intake of high-pesticide fruits and vegetables or choose organic versions. Low-pesticide products such as avocados, onions, sweet potatoes, broccoli, and oranges may also be good alternatives.

The Dirty Dozen are the foods you should only eat if they are organic. (New ones are on the EWG website each year.)[60]

DIRTY DOZEN

1. Strawberries
2. Spinach
3. Kale, collard, and mustard greens
4. Peaches
5. Pears

6. Nectarines

7. Apples

8. Grapes

9. Bell and hot peppers

10. Cherries

11. Blueberries

12. Green beans

DO YOU COMMONLY HAVE DIGESTIVE UPSETS?

If you have more digestive problems and aren't sure of what is causing them, looking into food sensitivity testing is a good idea. Constant inflammation in your digestive system not only affects your comfort but also your sleep and ability to absorb nutrients well.

Knowing your worst offending foods can help you avoid them and find other foods that might be new to you but you might enjoy. This is not a skin test, but one that tests your blood for reaction to foods. There are good options for this in Resources.

If your menstrual periods have been heavy for a long time, then anemia is something to investigate.

If you know that blood tests have shown low iron levels, hemoglobin, and hematocrit, then in addition to iron pills, or instead of, there are good food options to build blood.

Chicken liver or beef liver are very good sources of iron. Iron is stored in the liver for humans and animals, so cooking and eating grass-fed sourced liver will give your body iron, but also the other vitamins that are found in the liver.

Chicken liver:

- High in vitamin A, B vitamins, and folate

- Good source of protein with little to no carbohydrates

- Rich in minerals like selenium and iron

Beef liver:

- High in vitamin A, B vitamins, and copper

- Great source of high-quality protein
- Rich in minerals like iron, phosphorus, and zinc

Overall, beef liver has a richer nutritional profile compared to chicken liver, but both are excellent sources of nutrients. Beef liver has higher levels of B12, B2, B9, and A vitamins, as well as copper and choline.

Chicken liver, on the other hand, is denser in iron and selenium. Liver is also a great source of heme iron, which is the kind of iron that's most easily absorbed by the body and is essential for everyday function.[61]

Other sources of iron-rich foods are shellfish, legumes, spinach, red meat, pumpkin seeds, quinoa, turkey, broccoli, fish, and dark chocolate, to name a few.

If you are vegan or vegetarian, you will want to get a good digestible iron supplement.

The only caveat is if you have any family members who have been diagnosed with hemochromatosis. It is a genetic issue where you tend toward holding iron instead of moving it out of the liver and body. Normally, women aren't impacted by this until they have very light to no periods, as one way women "dump" iron is through the menstrual blood.

Men, however, don't have that option, and if they did have hemochromatosis or test with high levels of iron, then lowering iron content will be very important.

THE IMPORTANCE OF FOLATE

Another very important vitamin is folate. Folate is the natural form of vitamin B9, which is water-soluble and naturally found in many foods. On the other hand, folic acid is the synthetic form of vitamin B9 used in fortified foods and most dietary supplements. Folic acid must be converted into folate in the body to be effective.

The nutrient that is needed to help folic acid convert into folate is vitamin B12. It is required to convert folic acid to its active form, 5-methyltetrahydrofolate (5-MTHF), the form of folate that the body can use. Therefore, it is important to ensure adequate intake of both folic acid and vitamin B12 to maintain healthy levels of folate.

You might not think that something as simple as folate could make a difference in fertility, but I had a patient who was able to become pregnant but was having difficulty staying pregnant. She'd had a couple of miscarriages before she came to me for help. I talked to her about testing her B12 and folate levels, and after doing so, she learned that her levels were low due to having the MTHFR variant. Once she started taking a higher dosage of methylated folate, she was able to hold her next pregnancy.

Methylation is a simple biochemical process, and when optimal methylation occurs, it significantly impacts many biochemical reactions in the body that regulate the activity of the cardiovascular, neurological, reproductive, and detoxification systems.

It helps with DNA production, detoxification, estrogen, histamine, fat metabolism, cellular energy, and liver health, to name a few. This makes good methylation one big key to good health if you are taking good care of yourself!

Foods high in folate:

- Asparagus
- Avocado
- Broccoli, Brussels sprouts
- Green, leafy vegetables
- Legumes (peas, beans, lentils)
- Rice
- Liver (beef)
- Seafood
- Nuts and seeds

Seven specific nutrients can help the methylation cycle achieve optimal performance, even if an individual has the genetic mutation that slows down the methylation cycle.

- 5-MTHF (active folate)
- Methylcobalamin (active vitamin B12)
- Pyridoxal 5'-Phosphate (active vitamin B6)
- Riboflavin 5'-Phosphate (active vitamin B2)
- Magnesium (glycinate, taurine, malate, or a blend of these is preferable)

- Betaine (also known as trimethylglycine, it functions closely with choline, folic acid and B12)
- Vitamin D3

There are several different "cycles" in the body that need to work well for your longevity. Think of them like "little linked computers" that help each system function optimally. Without the essential vitamins and minerals, the computer's ability to work efficiently can be affected.

Each cycle needs different B vitamins or minerals, so eating a healthy diet and taking your prenatal is very important.

Homocysteine

Have homocysteine checked, as it is an important marker for how well you are methylating.

If levels are high, it can mean that you may not be absorbing folate (B9), B6, or B12. These are necessary for many body processes, so you need to ensure you are getting plenty in your diet and supplementation and avoiding foods that block or overutilize so you won't become depleted.

Vitamin B9 (folate), B6, and B12 can become depleted for various reasons.

Here are some causes of vitamin B deficiency:
- Dietary intake. Low dietary intake of vitamin B12, such as a low intake of animal-source foods, can cause vitamin B12 depletion. Vegetarians and vegans are at high risk of B12 deficiency.
- Malabsorption. The inability to release vitamin B12 from food, preventing its ability to be absorbed and utilized, which can be caused by low stomach acids that help digestion.
- Medications. Certain medications can deplete vitamin B9 (folic acid), such as antibiotics, antacids, and anti-inflammatory medications.
- Medical conditions. Certain medical conditions, such as Crohn's disease, celiac disease, HIV, and abusing alcohol, can prevent the body from absorbing B vitamins effectively, increasing the risk for deficiencies.
- Genetic factors. Some individuals can have a genetic code variation that affects a protein that transports vitamin B12 where need-

ed, such as the cells and tissues. Because of these genetic factors, some people might have more or less vitamin B12 in their blood.

Deficiencies in these B vitamins can lead to several different symptoms over time, such as anemia, fatigue, weakness, and nerve problems.

Maintaining adequate levels of these vitamins is important to reduce the risk of various diseases and conditions that can affect heart health, brain health, mental well-being, and more.

Glutathione

Glutathione is a super antioxidant that plays a key role in both male and female infertility. It helps preserve other antioxidants, including those present in both egg and sperm cells, aids in detoxification, and moderates the immune system.

Glutathione is present in both the male and female reproductive cells, and its level varies widely. Oxidative stress, caused by an imbalance between reactive oxygen species (ROS) and protective antioxidants, affects the entire reproductive lifespan of men and women.[62]

A common cause of male factor infertility is high levels of ROS biomarkers that can be detected in semen. When antioxidants are lacking, free radicals cause damage or death to cells, which can contribute to lower egg and sperm quality and infertility.

Numerous studies have shown that increasing the body's glutathione levels can increase egg, sperm, and embryo quality. For example, glutathione shields eggs from damage caused by oxidative stress during the formation of the follicles, and oocytes with higher levels of intracellular glutathione produce healthier and stronger embryos.

In women undergoing IVF, higher glutathione levels in a woman's follicle translated into increased fertilization rates. Low levels of follicular glutathione are associated with premature ovarian aging and lower fertilization rates. Glutathione also appears to be helpful in the regulation of chronic inflammation, which is a huge contributing factor to infertility.

Some symptoms common with glutathione deficiency are feeling tired (especially after any exercise), aches and pains in joints or muscles, brain fog, low immunity, poor sleep, and dry skin. It is present in almost all chronic diseases, including chronic stress, depression, and anxiety.

Deficiency of glutathione can be linked to poor diet, strenuous exercise, radiation exposure, smoking cigarettes or other tobacco products, alcohol consumption, pollution, exposure to pesticides or industrial chemicals, mold exposure, plastics, many cleaning supplies, and artificial fragrances.

Ways to increase glutathione:

1. It is important to detox your diet and eat a balanced diet containing sulfur-rich foods such as broccoli, garlic, and onions.

2. Some exercise, 20-30 minutes to sweat out toxins, is also helpful. (If 30 minutes makes you too tired, stick with 20 minutes.)

3. Eliminate alcohol and other toxic foods and substances.

4. Make sure you get enough sleep each night (seven to eight hours at least!)

5. Taking the supplements that help make glutathione can be less costly: Cysteine, glycine, and glutamate. Taking N-acetyl cysteine is a good precursor that is usually most needed. Other helpers are alpha lipoic acid, turmeric, whey protein, and vitamin C, or you could take liposomal glutathione.

WAYS TO INCREASE EGG QUALITY AND GOOD FERTILE MUCUS FOR OVULATION

A very important supplement to increase your egg quality is a prenatal with folate, not folic acid. This is also best when it has the most active forms of vitamins and minerals, as it will help it absorb much better. Avoid any prenatal blend containing fillers, such as magnesium stearate, sodium dioxide, and polyethylene glycol, whenever possible.

Other supplements to include:

- N-acetylcysteine—(antioxidant) reduces environmental and other toxins in eggs and sperm.
- Vitamin D3/K2—hormonal support, bone support.
- Omega 3s (DHA & EPA)—to lower inflammation.
- Myo & D-Chiro-Inositol—to help insulin receptivity (when HA1C is high or PCOS is present).
- Chaste Tree (Vitex)—supports ovulation, luteal phase, and progesterone levels.

- CoQ10—an antioxidant that can lessen chromosomal issues in eggs. (Stop if anxiety occurs.)

- Liposomal glutathione—a necessary antioxidant that can lessen chromosomal issues in the egg and cellular damage in the reproductive system and body.

- Choline and B12—(vegans and vegetarians especially need these as the highest quantities are in eggs and meat protein).

- DHEA—to increase ovarian reserve, but test hormones first to know if the level is deficient.

- Herbal blends—Different medicinal formulas are specific to the chief patterns. To be diagnosed and receive the right formula, we can set up a telemedicine consult, or you could visit a trusted local acupuncturist who specializes in herbal medicine.

I'm not suggesting that you take all these supplements. A comprehensive blood lab with a thorough hormone panel can reveal what is needed. Nutrient testing can also be done to cover all the vitamins and nutrients your body needs and your current levels. Then, you can make informed decisions on what to add supplementally.

Supporting your thyroid: Regardless of whether you have been diagnosed with hypothyroidism or Hashimoto's, there are supplements and medications that can help regulate your levels.

Selenium: found in prenatal supplements, 200 mcg a day is needed and normally in that amount in most prenatal supplements. For thyroid hormonal balance and more.

Zinc picolinate: zinc will typically be in all prenatal supplements, but often in low doses. Check to see if you're deficient with a zinc challenge or serum zinc testing.

A zinc challenge involves buying liquid zinc sulfate and putting a specified amount (listed on the bottle) into your mouth:

Response 1: No specific taste or other sensation is noticed after holding the solution in the mouth for up to 30 seconds. Indicates the need to supplement.

Response 2: No immediate taste is noted; however, after a few seconds, a slight taste develops, variously described as "dry," "mineral," "furry," or "sweet," which indicates that you need to supplement with zinc.

Magnesium: found to be deficient in most people and necessary for best functioning. (The best magnesium binders are glycinate, taurate, malate, and threonate.) The one that I use in my office combines the first three. If you have trouble sleeping or often feel muzzy-headed, the magnesium threonate is good as it passes through the blood-brain barrier.

If you are diagnosed with hypothyroidism, the following options are gluten-free:

Tirosint (synthetic T4): This is good when TSH levels are high, and gut issues are an issue.

Tirosint-SOL liquid ampules: It's free of gelatin. Tirosint-SOL is available in liquid single-dose ampules and only contains two inactive ingredients (glycerol and water).

Other gluten-free versions are Nature-Throid (T3 & T4), WP Thyroid, and Levothyroxine.

ACTION PLAN

- Make a copy of the "Dirty Dozen and Clean 15 Foods" to take to the grocery store. (This link is in Resources.)

- If you have digestive problems and aren't sure why, consider having food sensitivity testing and/or a thorough stool culture diagnostic test. It's good to add new foods to your diet regularly, as eating the same foods every day tends to cause sensitivity to those foods. Those sensitivities can cause inflammation in your digestive system.

- Clear out foods and items from your refrigerator and cabinets that are full of sugar, high fructose corn syrup, and alcohol, as well as fried and processed foods. These all deplete vitamins and minerals in your body and decrease glutathione levels.

- Before taking all vitamins listed, consider doing nutrient testing first to see what is needed. Tackling nutrient deficiencies first will make a good impact on your reproductive health.

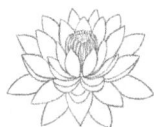

ASSISTED *Reproductive* THERAPIES (ART)

"Don't expect everyone to
understand your journey,

especially if they've never had
to walk your path."

—ANONYMOUS

Sometimes, after trying everything possible and being thoroughly tested, you're still not able to conceive. Looking for assisted reproductive therapies (ART) may be your best step.

If you've had all the testing mentioned in this book, have a diagnosis, changed your diet and supplemented for many months, made lifestyle changes for at least three months faithfully, and you're still having problems, then seeing a fertility specialist for a consult for ART is warranted, especially if you're near 40 years old.

Any process that involves a woman's egg or embryos (fertilized eggs) being handled falls under the umbrella term ART. Based on the CDC's 2021 Fertility Clinic Success Rates Report, approximately 238,126 patients had 413,776 ART cycles performed at 453 reporting clinics in the United States during 2021, resulting in 91,906 live births (deliveries of one or more living infants) and 97,128 live-born infants.[63]

Be sure to have all your lab information to help them figure out what the best option for pregnancy to occur is.

If you have an autoimmune condition, I suggest consulting with an autoimmune fertility specialist for the best results, as medications will be different.

INTRAUTERINE INSEMINATION: WHEN IS IT A GOOD IDEA?

The most common reasons for IUI are low sperm count or decreased sperm mobility. However, IUI may be selected as a fertility treatment for any of the following conditions as well:

- Unexplained infertility.
- A hostile cervical condition, including cervical mucus problems.
- Cervical scar tissue from past procedures may hinder the sperm's ability to enter the uterus.
- Ejaculation dysfunction.

WHEN IS HAVING AN IUI NOT A GOOD IDEA?

IUI is not recommended for the following patients:

- Women who have severe disease of the fallopian tubes.
- Women with a history of pelvic infections.
- Women with moderate to severe endometriosis.

The chance of becoming pregnant with multiples is increased if you take fertility medication when having IUI. There is also a small risk of infection after IUI.

"The success of IUI depends on several factors. If a couple has the procedure performed each month, success rates may reach as high as 20% per cycle depending on variables such as female age, the reason for infertility, and whether fertility drugs were used, among other variables."[64]

IVF—WHEN IT MIGHT BE NECESSARY

The most common type of ART is in vitro fertilization, commonly known as IVF. During IVF, a woman's eggs are removed from her body and fertilized in a lab. Once they've started to grow, the embryos are returned to the woman's uterus or frozen for use in the future.

The chances of pregnancy will depend on the age of a woman's eggs and many other factors particular to a couple, but on average, only 37 percent of assisted reproduction cycles for women under 35 result in live births. The chances of success decrease with age.[65]

Success rates vary among clinics, so it's important to discuss this with whatever fertility specialist or clinic you choose. Be sure to ask about live birth rates, not just pregnancy rates.

WHAT TO EXPECT WITH IVF

Dealing with infertility and undergoing IVF are stressful events, so it's no wonder that depression and anxiety are commonly reported among parents—particularly mothers—who are undergoing IVF.

The reason that stress, anxiety, and other mental health issues occur, besides taking this big step, is the medications do change things to help get you ready for egg retrieval. Since they'll want you to produce as many eggs as possible, several medications will be needed. Then, when they take the best embryo(s) to transfer, other medications will be used to ready your uterus for the transfer of the embryo. You'll never know how they would affect you individually, as everyone is different.

If you already have some mental health issues that you are dealing with, the medications could make them more severe, or you could find that you start to have issues while going through the IVF process.

Be sure to have a strong support system with family, friends, and possibly a therapist so you can be open about how you are feeling.

Although women have the most medical procedures associated with IVF, the whole process can be draining for hopeful dads as well. They may feel torn between dealing with their feelings of anxiety and stress and wanting to be "strong" for their partner.

SUCCESSFUL IVF—SMOOTH SAILING AHEAD?

Having a positive pregnancy test is, without a doubt, a joyous moment for couples who have undergone IVF. However, that test won't be the end of your worries.

This is not just with IVF or IUI, as you well know. Anytime pregnancy is achieved, there is always a waiting game full of hope and stress. Recurrent miscarriage has unfortunately made this "loop" agonizing while still maintaining hope that this will be the time that it works.

I've seen many patients go through this and know how heartbreaking it is when there is a first or second miscarriage. This is why I feel that it is so important to make changes to your diet and lifestyle, plus take anti-inflammatory and antioxidant supplements. If IVF is your best option, doing all of these steps will enhance your outcome!

If you decide on IVF in the United States, once the eggs have been fertilized, they will send the embryos for testing through a process called preimplantation genetic diagnosis (PGD).

PGD (PREIMPLANTATION GENETIC DIAGNOSIS)

During PGD, a single cell is removed from a developing embryo and tested for any genetic abnormalities, as they will implant only one or two healthy embryos. Most fertility specialists suggest that their patients do this to ensure the embryo(s) being transferred have the best chance of success.

MINI-IVF—IS THIS A BETTER OPTION?

Those qualifying for mini-IVF are patients with tubal factor infertility, couples who are not experiencing male factor infertility, women who are at greater risk of complications from injections used during conventional IVF, and individuals with a diminished ovarian reserve who have responded poorly to injections previously.

This method produces fewer embryos than conventional IVF. With conventional IVF, it is common for embryos to be discarded since they only want to implant a certain number. Some couples prefer to avoid this for religious or ethical reasons.

INCREASE YOUR CHANCE OF SUCCESS WITH ACUPUNCTURE

Recent research has illuminated the tangible benefits of acupuncture in IVF treatments. A systematic review and meta-analysis involving 4,757 participants found that acupuncture:

- Increased implantation rates by 28%

- Increased IVF clinical pregnancy rates by 33%
- Increased live birth rates by 33%
- Decreased the risk of biochemical pregnancies by 51%

The studies have shown that a series of acupuncture in the weeks leading up to retrieval/transfer and acupuncture immediately before and after the embryo transfer at the fertility clinic on the day of transfer can increase IVF/FET success.[66]

WHEN IS AN EGG OR SPERM DONOR A GOOD OPTION?

If you have a match in genetic issues or concerns over the results of egg or sperm quality, finding a donor could be a good option. Different agencies throughout the U.S. and the world work with those who are able to donate eggs or sperm.

The process can be daunting, so I've included a few sites in the Resources section of reputable places that you might want to work with.

If you do need to have ART, it's good to know the terms they use regularly.

Different assisted reproductive technology and their abbreviations:
- Intrauterine insemination (IUI)
- In vitro fertilization-embryo transfer (IVF-ET)
- Intracytoplasmic sperm injection (ICSI)
- Gamete intrafallopian transfer (GIFT)
- Preimplantation genetic testing (PGT)
- Zygote intrafallopian transfer (ZIFT)
- Frozen embryo transfer (FET)
- Donor conception (sperm, egg, embryos)

These techniques also apply to oocyte donation and surrogacy.

WHAT YOU SHOULD KNOW ABOUT SURROGACY

Surrogacy might be a hard decision for some and the only decision for others. If you've met with a specialist, had all the rigorous testing done with genetics, uterine receptivity, anatomical difficulties, and health history, and the results aren't good, it may be time to look into having a surrogate to bring your baby into your family.

Surrogacy is expensive. In the United States, the average journey costs $150,000, but the final cost can be much more or less depending on your circumstances. You are not required to work with a surrogacy agency, but complications often arise throughout the process. Most experts advise against going it alone.

A good surrogacy agency will ensure all the women carriers undergo health, criminal, financial, and psychological screenings before they're "matched." However, it's good to take the time to make sure it's a good fit. Your surrogacy "team" will probably include a reproductive endocrinologist, a lawyer, a psychologist, and an insurance specialist—interview several of each before hiring them.

Advancements in DNA testing have rendered the concept of "anonymous" egg and sperm donation obsolete, so decide what degree of openness you are comfortable with. In "gestational surrogacy," your surrogate and egg donor will be different. In "traditional surrogacy," the donor and surrogate are the same—meaning the carrier will be biologically related to the child.

ART AND THE BEST DIET PLAN

With the medications given during a standard IVF cycle, your diet is still critical for the best outcomes. Many IVFs can fail on the first attempt and subsequent IVFs as well if you don't address some of the underlying factors that impair conception and prevent miscarriages.

The best plan is to minimize inflammation and immune reactions as much as possible during the months before retrieval, before the transfer, and throughout the pregnancy.

Avoid the inflammatory categories of gluten (especially gliadin-based: wheat, rye, barley, and spelt), soy products, and dairy. Even the smallest amount of wheat in soy sauce can create inflammation. If you already know the foods that cause digestive or other problems, please avoid them as well.

ART AND SUPPLEMENTATION (WHEN ON MEDICATIONS)

During the pre-IVF timeframe, the supplements are not different from when you'd be trying naturally to conceive.

You should be taking:

- Prenatal vitamin with folate or methylfolate.
- CoQ10 (at least 300 mg a day) antioxidant to help egg quality.
- Omega-3 (3000 mg per day) to reduce inflammation and help blood circulation.
- Vitamin D3 (5000 IUs) Low levels can negatively impact your chance of conceiving through IVF.
- DHEA-S (25mg 1-2 times daily) if your DHEA levels and testosterone are both low.
- Myo-inositol (2gm a day) if fasting blood sugar levels are above 100 mg/dL and HA1C is above 5.6%.
- Tirosint or levothyroxine if TSH is above 2.5mU/L, FT4 is below 1.0ng/dL, FT3 is below 3pg/mL. Estrogen used before transfer to build the lining tends to lower thyroid hormone levels, so this needs to be checked more than once.

AUTOIMMUNE FERTILITY SPECIALISTS

If there are autoimmune challenges that are diagnosed and affecting conception or leading to recurrent miscarriages, then see a fertility specialist who is experienced in the treatment of your immune-related inflammation that is impacting conception and holding to term.

The book *Is Your Body Baby Friendly?* by the late Alan E. Beer, MD, has a lot of great information on the treatments he found most helpful in reducing an overactive immune system so conception and having a healthy child can become a reality.

His clinic in Los Gatos is now run by Raphael Stricker, MD, who utilizes Dr. Beer's protocols and testing methods.

For options, their website is: repro-med.net

You can also find help at: goivf.com/meet-the-experts

Unfortunately, the protocols used for immune-related issues can be expensive, so financially preparing for this is a good idea.

There are doctors worldwide who work with immune-related infertility. Search for "reproductive immunology doctors" near you.

ACTION PLAN

1. If you've tried everything mentioned in this book for at least four months, and it's still not happened for you and your husband, I highly recommend seeking out a fertility doctor who specializes in autoimmune-related issues.

2. Set up a telemedicine consultation if they're not local, and make sure you have all of your labs and tests available to fax to them.

3. If eggs and/or sperm are not testing well, talk to that doctor or investigate options for donor eggs and sperm and get a consultation with them.

4. If there are issues with genetics or anatomical problems, get a consultation with a surrogacy program and see what will work best for you.

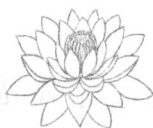

SUPPORTING *Your* FERTILITY

"Shout out to all of us fighting a battle
most people don't understand.

Keep hanging in there."

—ANONYMOUS

If you're like me and you like to skip to the end to get the basic wrap-up of the entire book before you even start reading the first chapter, I've got you covered. Here is a quick summary of five simple tips followed by a short list of what to avoid.

These are practical steps that you can take right now to support your reproductive wellness and dramatically increase the chances of getting to hold your newborn baby in your arms. I fully expect you to email me with the subject line: "We're pregnant!"

Until then …

1. Make sure that you buy a good prenatal multivitamin.

Don't buy a cheap brand, thinking they're all similar. That is far from the truth. I suggest finding a supplement with the following:

- Contains vitamins in their most absorbable forms, i.e., B6 as P5P, folate as methylfolate (not folic acid), methylcobalamin (B12), iron bisglycinate, magnesium glycinate, selenomethionine. Zinc picolinate needs to be higher than 15mg per day, and other B vitamins are more than 10mg. Vitamin D3 should have at least 1000 IUs.

- Make sure where it says "other ingredients" in small print that there are only a few. Do not buy supplements with polyethylene glycol, soybean oil, gluten, dairy, soy, eggs, nuts, or imitation colors and flavors.

2. Get good quality sleep.

I stress the importance of getting enough good sleep because it affects the following areas: sex hormones for ovulation and fertility, metabolism and endocrine system, and the immune system. Lack of sleep can cause inflammation, lower immunity, and increase stress and anxiety.

Go to bed early (before 10 p.m., if possible) and aim for eight hours of rested sleep. Step away from the TV and computer for at least an hour before bedtime. If sleep is difficult:

- Drink some Sleepy Time tea, chamomile, or another relaxing tea blend, and avoid caffeinated drinks after 3 p.m. You can also try 3mg of melatonin (it may cause mild anxiety, so if you already have anxiety, then avoid it) or try a CBD sleepy gummy.

- Stretching before bed can help blood flow and relaxation, especially when listening to soft, relaxing music.

- To lessen the disruption of "blue light" from the TV and computer screens, you can purchase "blue-light blocking" glasses.

- Magnesium malate (or threonate) can help with muscle relaxation for better sleep.

- Listen to soft music without lyrics. YouTube has a lot of calming musical options.

- Guided meditation (see the list of meditations on YouTube at the end if you don't already have one you love).

- Try using a sound machine, like Homedics, at night to encourage deeper sleep. Try steady rainfall, ocean waves, or other pink noises like leaves rustling in plants or trees.

3. Use fertile-friendly lubricant if the cervical mucus is scanty or absent.

If cervical mucus is not present or in too small an amount, using a fertility lubricant can help guide the sperm to its destination. The following are fertility-friendly choices.

- Yes Baby (all natural).
- Conceivable Plus.
- Baby Dance (no parabens).

If you're making enough natural lubrication with your partner, don't use any additional lubrication. Only use one of the "safe for conception sperm/vagina lubricates" if you have dryness. Clomid can tend to dry natural lubrication, and you'll want to use something to help the sperm travel upward if that is the case.

4. Get enough exercise.

This is important, as exercise helps:

- Enhance fertility by managing weight.
- Promote blood flow and hormonal balance.
- Counteract high stress.

Breaking a sweat can be very helpful in detoxification, too.

The key is moderation. Aim for 20-30 minutes of exercise that can bring on sweating. It's not quantity, it's quality. It can be brisk walking, hiking, swimming, dancing (even around the house), Zumba, calisthenics, or something that is fun for you.

5. Eat at least two healthy meals daily, preferably three.

Ensure each meal is balanced with protein, good fat, and a complex carb. (Example for breakfast: 2 eggs, ½ avocado, ½ cup berries.)

Try to eat your last meal no later than 6 p.m. to help you digest and sleep better. Doing this around your ovulation might make you feel more awake TTC.

WHAT TO AVOID

Do not douche. This washes away protective bacteria and will not help fertility.

If you notice an odor that you are trying to mask, get a pap smear and make sure that there's no infection taking place. If you know what the issue is, it can be treated.

Unfortunately, some things that cause this may get passed back and forth between you and your partner, so you both will need to be treated to stop it.

In addition, avoid the following:

- Caffeinated beverages—a 6-8 oz cup is okay per day, but better if avoided.
- Alcohol—avoidance is best.
- Nicotine—it's bad for you and the embryo, so please avoid this.
- Marijuana doesn't help fertility processes work well.
- NSAIDS (like ibuprofen) and recreational drugs—can impair ovulation.
- Antidepressants—unless necessary.

ACTION PLAN

1. Work on getting eight hours of quality sleep each night.
2. Stop adding chemicals like alcohol and recreational drugs to your body.
3. Make sure that any fertility lubricant you use is "baby-friendly."
4. Take a high-quality prenatal vitamin.
5. Find creative ways to reduce your daily stress.

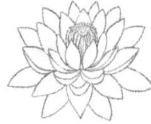

Afterword

As you come to the end of this book, I hope you feel empowered and uplifted by some of the stories of those who have faced unexplained infertility and found the answers they needed to start their families. Based on the symptoms you are dealing with, knowing which tests to ask for should help when you reach out to your OB/GYN or urologist (if male factor).

Having a complete diagnosis and plan is key. It's important to know your options for best health and treatment. If you need ART, you'll go into it knowing that it is your best option, as you and your partner have thoroughly tested.

Remember that you are not alone in your journey; there is always hope. With the help of traditional, holistic, and functional medicine and the support of loved ones, you, too, can overcome the challenges of infertility and fulfill your dream of having a baby.

Keep pushing forward, stay positive, and never give up on your dreams of a family.

Congratulations on taking the first step toward your future family, and best of luck on your journey!

REFERENCES

1   Louise Hay, *Heal Your Body: The Mental Causes for Physical Illness and the Metaphysical Way to Overcome Them* (Hay House Inc., 1995).

2   Mary Sabo, "Fertility and Chinese Herbs," FertilityIQ, accessed April 14, 2024, https://www.fertilityiq.com/fertilityiq/articles/fertility-and-chinese-herbs.

3   Taylor Graber, "Can Red Light Therapy Help Boost My Fertility?," ASAP IVs - IV Hydration Experts of San Diego, Phoenix, Scottsdale, San Francisco, November 16, 2022, https://www.asapivs.com/blog/2022/3/16/can-red-light-therapy-help-improve-my-fertility#:~:text=Red%20and%20near%20infrared%20light,natural%20pregnancies.

4   Katie Melville, "Nutrient-Depleted Soil: What It Means for Our Food," Chris Kresser, September 24, 2020, https://chriskresser.com/depletion-of-soil-and-what-can-be-done/.

5   Anket Sharma et al., "Worldwide Pesticide Usage and Its Impacts on Ecosystem ," SpringerLink, October 21, 2019, https://link.springer.com/article/10.1007/s42452-019-1485-1.

6   Kinga Skoracka et al., "Female Fertility and the Nutritional Approach: The Most Essential Aspects," Advances in nutrition (Bethesda, Md.), June 17, 2021, https://www.ncbi.nlm.nih.gov/pmc/articles/PMC8634384/.

7   Shuo Gu and Jianfeng Pei, "Innovating Chinese Herbal Medicine: From Traditional Health Practice to Scientific Drug Discovery," NIH National Library of Medicine, June 16, 2017, https://www.ncbi.nlm.nih.gov/pmc/articles/PMC5472722/#:~:text=Traditional%20Chinese%20Medicine%20has%20a,)%20(Reid%2C%201996

8   Tarek Gelbaya et al., "Definition and Epidemiology of Unexplained Infertility," Obstetrical & gynecological survey, February 2014, https://pubmed.ncbi.nlm.nih.gov/25112489/.

9   "Neurotransmitters: What They Are, Functions & Types," Cleveland Clinic, March 14, 2022, https://my.clevelandclinic.org/health/articles/22513-neurotransmitters.

10   Joanna Thompson, "No One Studied Menstrual Product Absorbency Realistically until Now," Scientific American, August 22, 2023, https://www.scientificamerican.com/article/no-one-studied-menstrual-product-absorbency-realistically-until-now/.

11   Dr. Amy Beckley, "Understanding Lufs with Guest Anna Saucier," Proov, April 16, 2020, https://proovtest.com/blogs/blog/lufs-anna-saucier.

12   "Infertility," World Health Organization, accessed January 23, 2024, https://www.who.int/health-topics/infertility.

13   Mark Mather, "The Decline in U.S. Fertility," PRB, July 18, 2012, https://www.prb.org/resources/the-decline-in-u-s-fertility/#:~:text=The%20decline%20in%20U.S.%20fertility%20has%20been%20driven%20primarily%20by,of%20women%20in%20their%2030s.

14   Liji Thomas, "Estradiol Measurement," News Medical Life Sciences, June 17, 2023, https://www.news-medical.net/health/Estradiol-Measurement.aspx.

15   Sarah Gavrizi, MD; Sushila Arya, MD; Jennifer Peck, PhD; Jennifer Knudtson, MD; Michael Diamond, MD; et al., "High-sensitivity C-reactive protein levels and pregnancy outcomes in women with unexplained infertility after ovarian stimulation with intrauterine insemination in a multicenter trial," NIH National

Library of Medicine, March 3, 2022, https://www.ncbi.nlm.nih.gov/pmc/articles/PMC8978106/#:~:text=Chronic%20inflammation%2C%20frequently%20assessed%20by,failures%20(2%2C%203)

16   CNY Fertility, "Benefits of Zinc for Sperm Quality and Overall Male Fertility," CNY Fertility, October 22, 2022, https://www.cnyfertility.com/zinc-and-sperm/#:~:text=Zinc%20and%20Male%20Fertility,-Zinc%20is%20a&text=The%20results%20of%20these%20studies,percentage%20of%20normal%20sperm%2-omorphology.

17   Tyler Bruce Garner et al., "Role of Zinc in Female Reproduction," NIH National Library of Medicine, May 2021, https://www.ncbi.nlm.nih.gov/pmc/articles/PMC8599883/#:~:text=Zinc%20is%20a%20critical%20component,is%20ready%20to%20undergo%20maturation

18   Gerson Weiss et al., "Inflammation in Reproductive Disorders," Reproductive sciences (Thousand Oaks, Calif.), February 2009, https://www.ncbi.nlm.nih.gov/pmc/articles/PMC3107847/.

19   "Autoimmunity," Wikipedia, January 17, 2024, https://en.wikipedia.org/wiki/Autoimmunity.

20   Alan E. Beer, Julia Kantecki, and Jane Reed, *Is Your Body Baby-Friendly?: Unexplained Fertility, Miscarriage & IVF Failure Explained & Treated* (AJR Publishing, 2006).

21   Lara Pellegrinelli, "5 Causes of Unexplained Infertility," Experience Life, August 30, 2017, https://experiencelife.lifetime.life/article/5-causes-of-unexplained-infertility/.

22   "Thrombophilia," Pacific Fertility Center Los Angeles, accessed March 11, 2024, https://www.pfcla.com/fertility-101/causes-of-miscarriage/thrombophilia/.

23   "Polycystic Ovary Syndrome (PCOS)," Johns Hopkins Medicine, February 28, 2022, https://www.hopkinsmedicine.org/health/conditions-and-diseases/polycystic-ovary-syndrome-pcos#:~:text=Key%20points,%2C%20infertility%2C%20and%20weight%20again.

24   Sarah Jayawardene, "Insulin Resistance and Fertility: Everything You Need to Know," Veri, accessed March 9, 2024, https://www.veri.co/learn/insulin-resistance-and-infertility.

25   Dania Al-Jaroudi et al., "Non-Alcoholic Fatty Liver Disease in Infertile Women with Polycystic Ovarian Syndrome: A Prospective Series," ClinMed International Library, March 20, 2017,

https://clinmedjournals.org/articles/ijwhw/international-journal-of-womens-health-and-wellness-ijwhw-3-047.php?jid=ijwhw#ref7.

26   Suneeta Senapati, "Managing Endometriosis Leading to Infertility," Pennmedicine.org, April 10, 2019, https://www.pennmedicine.org/research-at-penn/online-research-interviews/managing-endometriosis-leading-to-infertility.

27   G Willy Davila, "Endometriosis Workup," Medscape, July 18, 2023, https://emedicine.medscape.com/article/271899-workup.

28   See the Resources section at the end of the book for Environmental Working Group (EWG) for the list of foods in each category.

29   "Hydrosalpinx," Cleveland Clinic, November 11, 2022, https://my.clevelandclinic.org/health/diseases/24437-hydrosalpinx#symptoms-and-causes.

30   Goswami Binita et al., "Correlation of Prolactin and Thyroid Hormone Concentration with Menstrual Patterns in Infertile Women," Journal of reproduction

& infertility, October 2009, https://www.ncbi.nlm.nih.gov/pmc/articles/
PMC3719326/.

31   Izabella Wentz, *Hashimoto's Protocol: A 90-Day Plan for Reversing Thyroid Symptoms and Getting Your Life Back* (New York, NY: HarperOne, an imprint of HarperCollins Publishers, 2017).

32   Alan R McNeil and Phoebe E Stanford, "Reporting Thyroid Function Tests in Pregnancy," The Clinical biochemist. Reviews, November 2015, https://www.ncbi.nlm.nih.gov/pmc/articles/PMC4758281/#:~:text=The%20American%20Endocrine%20Society%20also,in%20the%20second%20and%20third.

33   George Elhomsy, "Antithyroid Antibody," Medscape, June 2, 2022, https://emedicine.medscape.com/article/2086819-overview#a1?form=fpf.

34   Alan E. Beer, Julia Kantecki, and Jane Reed, *Is Your Body Baby-Friendly?: Unexplained Fertility, Miscarriage & IVF Failure Explained & Treated* (AJR Publishing, 2006).

35   "MTHFR Gene, Folic Acid, and Preventing Neural Tube Defects," Centers for Disease Control and Prevention, June 15, 2022, https://www.cdc.gov/ncbddd/folicacid/mthfr-gene-and-folic-acid.html#:~:text=MTHFR%20gene%20variants%20are%20common.&text=In%20fact%2C%20there%20are%20more,who%20do%20not.

36   Kim Smith-Whitley, "Reproductive Issues in Sickle Cell Disease," ScienceDirect, December 4, 2014, https://www.sciencedirect.com/science/article/pii/S000649712039604X.

37   Kim Smith-Whitley, Reproductive issues in sickle cell disease, December 4, 2014, https://pubmed.ncbi.nlm.nih.gov/25472967/.

38   Kristen Wendell, "Sickle Cell Anemia," Michigan State University The Oncofertility Consortium, September 24, 2014, https://oncofertility.msu.edu/non-malignant-conditions/sickle-cell-anemia/.

39   "How Does Cystic Fibrosis Affect Reproductive Health and Fertility?," Cystic Fibrosis16, August 2019, https://cystic-fibrosis.com/infertility.

40   Jianli Sun, Melissa A. Harrington, and Ben Porter, "Sex Difference in Spinal Muscular Atrophy Patients – Are Males More Vulnerable?," Journal of Neuromuscular Diseases, September 8, 2023, https://content.iospress.com/articles/journal-of-neuromuscular-diseases/jnd230011.

41   Saniya Rattan et al., "Exposure to Endocrine Disruptors during Adulthood: Consequences for Female Fertility," The Journal of endocrinology, June 2017, https://www.ncbi.nlm.nih.gov/pmc/articles/PMC5479690/.

42   Amy Ratner, "Celiac Disease Reproductive Health Heartbreak," Beyond Celiac, July 6, 2018, https://www.beyondceliac.org/research-news/celiac-disease-reproductive-health-heartbreak/.

43   Justine Bold and Kamran Rostami, "Non-Coeliac Gluten Sensitivity and Reproductive Disorders," Gastroenterology and hepatology from bed to bench, 2015, https://www.ncbi.nlm.nih.gov/pmc/articles/PMC4600520/.

44   Andrew C Dukowicz, Brian E Lacy, and Gary M Levine, "Small Intestinal Bacterial Overgrowth: A Comprehensive Review," Gastroenterology & hepatology, February 2007, https://www.ncbi.nlm.nih.gov/pmc/articles/PMC3099351/.

45   Gal Wald et al., "Assessing the Clinical Value of the Kruger Strict Morphology Criteria Over the World Health Organization Fourth Edition Criteria," NIH National Library of Medicine, April 19, 2021, https://www.ncbi.nlm.nih.gov/pmc/articles/

PMC8267392/#:~:text=In%20the%20fifth%20edition%20of,spermatozoa%20
are%20considered%20morphologically%20abnormal

46   Kristin Brogaard, "What Is Sperm Morphology in My Semen Analysis Results?,"
Path Fertility, November 16, 2023, https://pathfertility.com/what-is-sperm-
morphology-in-my-semen-analysis-results-2/#:~:text=4%25%20is%20normal%20
based%20on,male%20has%20abnormally%20shaped%20sperm.

47   "Endocrine Disruptors," National Institute of Environmental Health Sciences,
February 6, 2024, https://www.niehs.nih.gov/health/topics/agents/endocrine.

48   Kimberly Holland, "Signs and Symptoms of High Estrogen," Healthline, January
30, 2024, https://www.healthline.com/health/high-estrogen.

49   Michael Schulster, Aaron M Bernie, and Ranjith Ramasamy, "The Role of
Estradiol in Male Reproductive Function," Asian journal of andrology, February 23,
2016, https://www.ncbi.nlm.nih.gov/pmc/articles/PMC4854098/.

50   "Erectile Dysfunction (ED): Symptoms, Causes, Diagnosis, and Treatment,"
Healthline, November 29, 2023, https://www.healthline.com/health/erectile-
dysfunction.

51   "High Blood Sugar and Male Infertility," Your Fertility, January 7, 2019, https://
www.yourfertility.org.au/high-blood-sugar-and-male-infertility.

52   Xiang Li et al., "Effects of Folic Acid Plus Zinc Supplements on the Sperm
Characteristics and Pregnancy Outcomes of Infertile Men: A systemic Review and
Meta-Analysis," NIH National Library of Medicine, July 13, 2023, https://www.ncbi.
nlm.nih.gov/pmc/articles/PMC10395467/

53   Jamin Brahmbhatt, "Does Smoking Weed Affect Sperm Count? Here's What
Fertility Science Says," Fatherly, September 13, 2019, https://www.fatherly.com/
health/smoking-weed-and-sperm-fertility-science.

54   Joseph Pizzorno, "Environmental Toxins and Infertility," Integrative medicine
(Encinitas, Calif.), April 17, 2018, https://www.ncbi.nlm.nih.gov/pmc/articles/
PMC6396757/#:~:text=The%20worst%20fertility%20disrupters%20are,air%20
pollutants%20seriously%20damage%20fertility.

55   Diala El Khoury et al., "Updates on the Effect of Mycotoxins on Male
Reproductive Efficiency in Mammals," NIH Library of Medicine, September 2019,
https://www.ncbi.nlm.nih.gov/pmc/articles/PMC6784030/

56   Joseph Pizzorno, "Environmental Toxins and Infertility," Integrative medicine
(Encinitas, Calif.), April 17, 2018, https://www.ncbi.nlm.nih.gov/pmc/articles/
PMC6396757/#:~:text=The%20worst%20fertility%20disrupters%20are,air%20
pollutants%20seriously%20damage%20fertility.

57   Sohyae Lee, Jin-young Min, and Kyoung-bok Min, "Female Infertility Associated
With Lead and Cadmium," NIH National Library of Medicine, March 17, 2020,
https://www.ncbi.nlm.nih.gov/pmc/articles/PMC7084729/#B9-ijerph-17-01794

58   Yu-Han Chiu, Paige Williams, and Matthew Gillman, "Pesticide Residue Intake
and Assisted Reproductive Technology Outcomes," JAMA Internal Medicine,
January 1, 2018, https://jamanetwork.com/journals/jamainternalmedicine/
fullarticle/2659557.

59   Yu-Han Chiu, "Pesticides in Produce Linked with Reduced Fertility in Women,"
Harvard T.H. Chan School of Public Health, October 30, 2017, https://www.hsph.
harvard.edu/news/hsph-in-the-news/pesticides-produce-fertility-women/.

60   "Dirty DozenTM Fruits and Vegetables with the Most Pesticides," EWG's 2023
Shopper's Guide to Pesticides in Produce | Dirty Dozen, accessed February 18, 2024,
https://www.ewg.org/foodnews/dirty-dozen.php.

61   Kathryn Brunk, "Chicken Liver vs. Beef Liver: Battle of Two Superfoods," Doctor Kiltz, January 3, 2022, https://www.doctorkiltz.com/chicken-liver-beef-liver/.

62   Oyewopo Adeoye et al., "Review on the Role of Glutathoine on Oxidative Stress and Infertiity," PMC PubMed Central, Jan.-March 2018, https://www.ncbi.nlm.nih.gov/pmc/articles/PMC5844662/.

63   "2021 Assisted Reproductive Technology Fertility Clinic and National Summary Report," CDC.gov, 2021, https://www.cdc.gov/art/reports/2021/pdf/Report-ART-Fertility-Clinic-National-Summary-H.pdf.

64   "Intrauterine Insemination: IUI," American Pregnancy Association, June 13, 2022, https://americanpregnancy.org/getting-pregnant/intrauterine-insemination/#:~:text=What%20is%20IUI%27s%20Success%20Rate,were%20used%2C%20among%20other%20variables.

65   Kelly Burch, "12 IVF Truths No One Tells You About," CCRM Fertility, April 27, 2022, https://www.ccrmivf.com/news-events/ivf-truths/.

66   Menghao Xu, Mengdi Zhu, and Cuihong Zheng, "Effects of Acupuncture on Pregnancy Outcomes in Women Undergoing in Vitro Fertilization: An Updated Systematic Review and Meta-Analysis - Archives of Gynecology and Obstetrics," SpringerLink, July 12, 2023, https://link.springer.com/article/10.1007/s00404-023-07142-1.

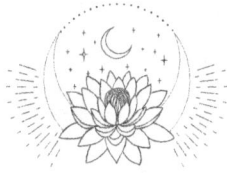

THE

Journey

CONTINUES

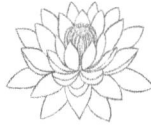

HOW TO GET
MORE *Help*

Many of my patients love to get a jumpstart when it comes to priming their body for conception, and that means having a clear starting point.

That's why I always recommend starting with my complimentary **Simple 2-Week Body Reset** guide, also available at:

ShellyTompkins.com

With this free guide, you'll give your body a chance to clear out all the unhealthy foods and substances in your diet that lead to fatigue, hormonal imbalances, nutrient deficiencies, and excessive toxins, which can have a negative impact on your health and fertility. You and your baby deserve a fresh starting point!

ADDITIONAL RESOURCES

Most Popular Links:

Two-Week Fertility Body Reset & Detox Plan | shellytompkins.com

Castor Oil Pack Directions for Fertility | bit.ly/43b3LYC

EWG Dirty Dozen and Clean 15 Food List | ewg.org

Free Printable BBT Chart | bit.ly/3V6IGg8

Healthy Skincare | ewg.org/skindeep

Safe Fertility Lubricants:

Certified Organic Personal Lubricants by AH! YES | ahyes.org

Duo Fertility Lubricant Bundle | conceiveplus.com

Baby Dance Fertility Lubricant | fairhavenhealth.com

To find an egg donor, surrogate, or IVF clinic, see the suggestions below:

GoStork | gostork.com

Extraordinary Conceptions | extraconceptions.com

Hatch | hatch.us

You can also do a Google search for mini-IVF clinics near you.

Yoni Steaming Resources:

Castor Oil Packs & Yoni Steaming Herbs | shellytompkins.com/shop

Yoni Steaming Stools | etsy.com/market/yoni_steam_seat

DIY Yoni Steaming Directions:

1. Pour 10 cups of filtered water (purified water is best) into a large pot with a lid.

2. Put the prescribed herbs into the water and bring the water to a low boil.

3. Turn the heat off, leave the lid on, and let it steep for 5 minutes more.

4. Double-check the water temperature before use; if it is too hot, let it set for 20 seconds and recheck until it feels comfortably warm.

5. Pour 3-4 cups of herbal water into a stainless steel bowl (not plastic) in the toilet.

6. Check once more before sitting on the toilet seat to make sure that it will be comfortable.

7. Remove your underwear and sit on the seat over the steam.

8. Have a nice, guided meditation journal ready, and have some relaxing music playing.

9. Make sure you are warm. Use a warm blanket to cover your legs and wear socks.

10. Plan for about 10 minutes the first time you steam, and see how you feel.

11. If you feel good with 10 minutes, plan to do these a couple days before ovulation.

12. Beware! Never steam when you are on your period or when irregularly bleeding.

As always, if you need updated links or additional help,
reach out to me at:

ShellyTompkins.com

ACKNOWLEDGMENTS

To my wonderful husband, Jeff, whose support and encouragement helped tremendously in completing this labor of love.

I want to thank my dad for his encouragement to follow in his footsteps, who passed away in 2016 and is very missed. He was a Homeopath, Naturopath, and Doctor of Acupuncture and Oriental Medicine. With everything that I have learned in my studies of functional medicine and my work with my patients, I realize that he was ahead of his time with the underlying factors that cause disease. I learned so much from him and hope to make him proud of me in the afterlife. I am grateful to my mom for the support and love she has given me throughout my life and in my holistic practice.

I'm very grateful to my editing team, Lori Lynn and Mary Rembert, who helped shape this book and kept me going with their encouragement, talent, and humor. Also, my publisher, Shanda Trofe, who was so helpful with her insights throughout this process, and Esther Moody, who did the beautiful artistry for this book's design.

I want to thank all of my teachers in both Chinese Medicine and Functional Medicine, especially Alex Tiberi, Giovanni Macioccia, Jane Lyttleton, Jeffrey Yuen, Bob Flaws, Ben Lynch, Datis Kharrazian, and Claudia Citzkovitz, who helped stretch my thinking of how the body works and the best ways to give treatment.

I want to thank those close friends who believed in me and encouraged me to write this book.

I'd also like to thank all the patients that I have worked with over the years who have helped me understand their fertility struggles and let me be part of their healing journey to have a family.

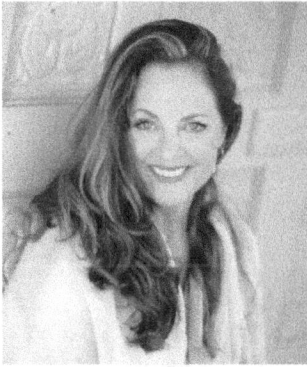

ABOUT THE *Author*

Shelly Weber-Tompkins, L.Ac, CFMP, is a renowned Integrative Wellness Expert, Licensed Acupuncturist, and Certified Functional Medicine Practitioner specializing in women's health, fertility, and pregnancy, as well as postpartum and immune conditions.

She has been in private practice for over 35 years and was a professor at Pacific College of Health Sciences (then PCOM) for 24 years. At PCOM, she taught courses in OB/GYN, integrating them with Traditional Chinese Medicine (TCM) and treatment for infertility in couples. She served as a private practitioner there as well as a clinical supervisor.

Shelly also had the privilege of working with the midwives at UCSD's Perlman Clinic in San Diego. She practiced there for four years, where she treated women for infertility, perinatal, and postpartum-related issues while running a private practice in San Diego.

Throughout her career, Shelly has helped thousands of families in their fertility journey at her clinic, Fertile Lifestyle Acupuncture and Integrative Medicine. She is well known for her ability to help couples overcome their fertility obstacles and then help them throughout their pregnancy and postpartum recovery.

Shelly is currently in practice in her clinic in San Diego, CA, and is passionate about her continued studies in Asian Medicine and integrative medicine therapies, finding them great tools for finding deeper, not-so-obvious solutions. She also shares this knowledge and expertise on podcasts and speaking engagements. All inquiries for podcast appearances and speaking can be sent to shelly@shellytompkins.com.

Shelly loves spending time with her husband, Jeff, and their new cat. Shelly enjoys hiking, tennis, playing pool, visiting her mom and sister's family, and spending quality time with her close friends.

You can find Shelly online at **ShellyTompkins.com.**

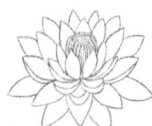

NEXT STEPS

Whether you have been struggling with infertility or are just getting started on your journey and want to set yourself up for success, I would love to help you.

I am available for in-person and telehealth sessions, but the best place to start is with a free 20-minute consultation.

Once I get to know you and your needs, I'll lay out a clear plan of action tailored specifically to you and your unique situation so that you know which next steps to take.

To book your FREE 20-minute consultation, go here:

ShellyTompkins.com